Intentional Health

Intentional Health

DETOXIFY, NOURISH AND REJUVENATE YOUR BODY INTO BALANCE

• • • • • • •

Dr Chiti Parikh

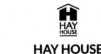

HAY HOUSE

Carlsbad, California • New York City
London • Sydney • New Delhi

Published in the United Kingdom by:
Hay House UK Ltd, The Sixth Floor, Watson House,
54 Baker Street, London W1U 7BU
Tel: +44 (0)20 3927 7290; Fax: +44 (0)20 3927 7291; www.hayhouse.co.uk

Published in the United States of America by:
Hay House Inc., PO Box 5100, Carlsbad, CA 92018-5100
Tel: (1) 760 431 7695 or (800) 654 5126
Fax: (1) 760 431 6948 or (800) 650 5115; www.hayhouse.com

Published in Australia by:
Hay House Australia Ltd, 18/36 Ralph St, Alexandria NSW 2015
Tel: (61) 2 9669 4299; Fax: (61) 2 9669 4144; www.hayhouse.com.au

Published in India by:
Hay House Publishers India, Muskaan Complex, Plot No.3, B-2,
Vasant Kunj, New Delhi 110 070
Tel: (91) 11 4176 1620; Fax: (91) 11 4176 1630; www.hayhouse.co.in

Indexer: J S Editorial LLC
Cover design: Jason Gabbert Design
Interior design: Joe Bernier
Interior photos/illustrations: Fendi Kurniawan and Zuhaib Naqvi

A catalogue record for this book is available from the British Library.

Tradepaper ISBN: 978-1-83782-095-5
E-book ISBN: 978-1-83782-219-5
Audiobook ISBN: 978-1-83782-218-8

This product uses papers sourced from responsibly managed forests. For more information, see www.hayhouse.co.uk.

Printed and bound by CPI Group (UK) Ltd, Croydon CR0 4YY

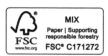

To my grandmother, whose unconditional love and wisdom have been a guiding light in my life

CONTENTS

Introduction ix

Part I: Charting the Path
Chapter 1   Your Health Intention 3

Part II: Seven Ancient Secrets
Chapter 2   The Circadian Rhythm 13
Chapter 3   The Good Bacteria... 39
Chapter 4   The Digestive Fire 61
Chapter 5   The Root Cause.. 83
Chapter 6   The Anti-Aging Detox 109
Chapter 7   The Mind-Body Connection.............................. 131
Chapter 8   The Breath of Life.. 151

Part III: Sustaining Intentional Health
Chapter 9   The 28-Day Reset.. 173
Chapter 10 The 20-Minute Daily Ritual 201

Endnotes.. 207
Index 225
Acknowledgments 232
About the Author 233

INTRODUCTION

As the co-founder and executive director of Integrative Health and Wellbeing at Weill Cornell, a 15,000-square-foot, state-of-the-art healing oasis on the Upper East Side of Manhattan, New York, I know my patients often wait months for an appointment. They arrive with high hopes of finally receiving a proper diagnosis. Most of them have been suffering from their ailments for months—or even years. During this time, each has been passed around from specialist to specialist like a hot potato. Every expert zooms in on the one symptom or body part that falls under their purview.

Western doctors are trained to record a set of symptoms, generate a list of diagnoses that match them, and write a prescription. In other words, they're taught to match every ill to a pill. This approach assumes all patients with the same symptoms or diagnosis will benefit from the same medication. That might work when trying to fix a car or a computer, but we're far more than just the sum of our body parts. We can't be reduced to such simplistic labels.

I've been a patient myself, so I know how daunting the process of obtaining health care can be. Usually, we get only 10 or 15 minutes with a doctor. How can any patient explain everything they've experienced in that amount of time? Meanwhile, physicians are often tasked with reviewing years of medical records, performing an exam, providing an assessment, and creating a treatment plan within that same 10 or 15 minutes. That isn't even enough time to get through an episode of a TV show, let alone address the most precious thing we have—our health.

As a result, most people feel betrayed by their bodies. This happens despite the fact that we live in an age when we have access to a seemingly infinite amount of information at our fingertips. It's ironic that we still feel lost when it comes to our health. This is why, when I started my practice, I made a promise to myself that

I would give every patient the time they deserved. Now I have the privilege and the pleasure of practicing integrative medicine, which prioritizes being fully present to have a conversation with, listen to, and connect with my patients.

Of course, everyone who enters the field of medicine does so with these aims in mind. I don't remember anything in the medical school brochures about spending hours on the computer or arguing with insurance companies. We all start out with the right intentions, but somehow we become lost in the chaos of our health-care system. Unfortunately, we also get swept up in the way Western medicine defines health.

EAST AND WEST

Western medicine essentially defines *health* as "the mere absence of disease," while Eastern medicine equates health to a balance between our body, mind, and spirit. It considers the ups and downs in life and provides a practical approach to maintaining equanimity through it all.

When we take only the physical symptoms into account, we miss the forest for the trees. No wonder the World Health Organization now defines *health* as "a state of complete physical, mental and social well-being and not merely the absence of disease or infirmity."[1] I would go so far as to say that *health is about living a life full of energy and manifesting your true potential, with your body as your best ally.*

People often ask me, "Do you treat hormone issues, anxiety, stress, gastrointestinal issues, or autoimmune conditions?" My answer is: *I treat people, not diseases or symptoms.* We have to consider the psychological, social, environmental, and spiritual components that make each person unique. And we must strive to balance all these aspects of who we are.

In my personal and professional life, I always strive for balance. Every day, I work smart and hard to nourish, detoxify, and rejuvenate my body to stay vital and healthy. I share this knowledge with my patients to help them balance their hectic modern lives as well.

Many of them are surprised to find out that health doesn't have to cost a lot of money or time. In fact, contrary to what the multibillion-dollar health and wellness industry would have us believe, staying healthy is free and easy.

I firmly believe that everything needed to live a long, healthy life is programmed into our DNA. The evidence is the determined survival and evolution of humankind itself. Each of our bodies carries within it the knowledge of how to survive and thrive regardless of the challenges we face. Tapping into this inner intelligence can be a powerful force for health.

It's largely a matter of following some important principles that the sages in Eastern medicine traditions have known for generations. If we do that, the body is often capable of remaining in balance and healing itself. These principles are the fundamental building blocks for our body and mind to work effortlessly. They're the keys to attaining maximum results from everything we do to maintain health, such as making diet, exercise, and lifestyle changes.

And now, modern Western science is starting to catch up and validate the erudition behind this sage wisdom. Why rely on just the last 50 years of science, when we can expand our tool kit to include healing traditions that have evolved over hundreds, if not thousands, of years?

Using these age-old principles, you can take steps every day to ensure your vitality and health. While a book can never substitute for a doctor's care or provide an individualized assessment of what's going on in *your* body, the best patients are proactive and learn as much as they can about maintaining their health. No doctor will ever know your body, mind, or spirit as well as you do, but they can offer you better care when you actively participate in your health journey—with intention.

In that spirit, on these pages, I will combine a five-thousand-year history rooted in time-tested, ancient traditions with cutting-edge science. I'll provide steps you can take to bring your body into a healthier state of balance, which will give you a better chance of warding off disease. This approach has helped my patients not only live longer lives but also live with more energy, less pain, and renewed confidence.

Never underestimate the power of your body (with the help of your mind and spirit) to heal itself. The human body is truly a miraculous invention. It's capable of so much more than most of us give it credit for. If you've ever doubted that, let me persuade you with the story of the yogi who lived to be 185 years old.

THE 185-YEAR-OLD YOGI

Having grown up in India, I had heard a bit about this sage, who was born there in the 1700s and died on October 12, 1955. However, I wasn't aware that a detailed account of his life had been published by one of his disciples until it popped up as a recommendation one day while I was searching for medical books. I still have no explanation why, but I was happy to find a copy.

As you can imagine, the life of this yogi was full of mystery and supernatural occurrences that would dissuade any "rational" person from believing in them. But I had met my own share of yogis with uncanny abilities that I couldn't explain through any scientific means. Our limited understanding of these phenomena is likely because science hasn't yet caught up with them. Yet, when most of us encounter something that's beyond our comprehension, we automatically label it as fake. For example, imagine if someone handed you the latest iPhone and a self-driving car in the 1980s. You would have thought they were props from a movie like *Back to the Future*. But in our lifetime, these fictional artifacts are now part of our daily life.

So, why does the story of a 185-year-old yogi raise eyebrows? If our current science can enable us to live to about 100, why can't the future (or perhaps our past) hold the key to a 185-year lifespan?

This particular yogi was born into royalty but gave up his title and lavish lifestyle to spend the rest of his life in the Himalayan Mountains. He walked thousands of miles on foot with only a loincloth to cover his body while carrying a pitcher of water as his companion. His body had to endure the harshest of climates, prolonged fasts, and assaults from wild animals.

As if that weren't enough, he spent decades performing severe penances that far surpassed what we think of as the boundaries of the human body. For a decade at a time, he took the vow of silence, didn't sit down, and even held up his arm for longer than 12 years! Even today, you will come across such yogis wandering the shores of the holy Ganges River.

Well past turning 100 and for a period of 12 years, the yogi spent entire hot Indian summers meditating in the direct sun in the afternoons. In the bitter winter, he meditated in the middle of the night while cold water was poured on him.

These actions weren't a punishment for sins. They were meant to push the limits of his body to help him gain control of both his mind and physicality, thus aiding his spiritual progress. Undisturbed by physical pain or mental chatter, this yogi and others like him were able to turn inward with complete focus and surrender. They were masters of their minds, but their bodies were still susceptible to wear and tear, so they figured out the science of rejuvenation to keep their bodies vital while they continued their

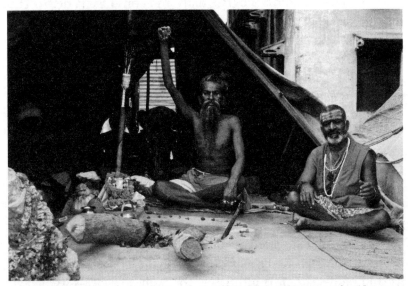

Amar Bharti: Indian man who has been holding his right arm up for 45 years

pursuit of eternal truth. They often went without food, especially when they meditated for months at a time in remote caves in sub-zero temperatures. They could do so by mastering control of their metabolism through their intense yoga practice.

As the 185-year-old yogi turned 90, he felt the limitations of his physical body. During this time, he met another yogi who possessed the knowledge of an ancient technique called *kaya kalpa*. (*Kaya* means "body," and *kalpa* means "transformation.") This technique is meant only for advanced yogis, as it helps them rejuvenate their bodies by undoing the afflictions brought on by aging.

Kaya kalpa is rigorous, and only someone with exceptional mental strength and extreme tolerance for physical discomfort can handle it. A yogi who can walk around with his arm raised above his head for a decade, however, certainly meets the criteria.

To prepare one's body for the kaya kalpa, a yogi has to go through initial preparatory cleanses, like the process of *pancha-karma* detoxification. After that, he retreats to a cell specially constructed for the process.

He spends the entire duration of the treatment in that windowless cell, which does not allow anyone in except the physician who checks on his progress daily and administers herbs. The hut the old yogi used was designed not even to let in any light or sound. The environment was intended to mimic being in a mother's womb, allowing for total sensory deprivation. Most of us would lose our minds if we were subjected to these conditions even for a day. Imagine being in solitary confinement in a dark room, subsisting on cow's milk and herbs, and spending all of your time meditating for a year! This might be a yogi's dream, but for most of us, it's a claustrophobic nightmare.

These steps do seem rather extreme, but that is what it takes to unlock the fountain of youth. The most important concept of this process is allowing the inner intelligence of the body to function as it was meant to. There are many myths about magical herbs and potions that are often credited for the incredible results of this process. However, herbs can only assist the body to help detoxify and rejuvenate. It is ultimately the body that heals itself. The yogi's task is to allow the body to do its job by minimizing distraction and conserving energy through complete sensory deprivation, fasting, and meditating.

This yogi's kaya kalpa treatment at the age of 90 lasted almost a year, after which he emerged full of vitality and free of diseases, not to mention with new teeth, hair, and skin. He was then able to continue his intense practices with the body of a 30-year-old.

During his lifetime, he underwent this rejuvenation process three times—at the ages of 90, 150, and 165. It allowed him to turn back the clock enough to continue his spiritual practice.

Of course, I don't expect myself or anyone else I know to endure all of that—not even for the benefit of living 185 years. But the story of this yogi indicates that our bodies are capable of much more than we've realized. And the more I've researched the story of the 185-year-old, the more science I've found behind it. It isn't the "mystical miracle" one would expect. This science is also not unique to Indian yogis. It's found in many parts of the world and has been used by serious spiritual seekers for eons.

For example, the Ayurvedic detoxification called panchakarma mentioned above, which the yogi practiced to prepare his body for kaya kalpa, is accessible to anyone. We can do it for a much shorter time and without the rigorous requirements the yogi endured.

Meanwhile, kaya kalpa itself is a highly specialized method of activating stem cells, which are special cells we all carry. They can become practically any kind of cell, such as the ones in our heart, brain, bones, muscles, and skin. They're often activated when our body needs to replace cells that have aged or have been damaged. If we want to remain young and healthy, these are the cells we need to activate.

The yogis simply figured out a way to unlock the potential of stem cells. They were able to transform them to reverse aging and breathe vitality back into the body. These multipotent cells, which can transform into any cell, whether it's for hair, skin, teeth, or an organ, hold tremendous potential because they can be used to cure all kinds of diseases like cancer, heart disease, stroke, and Parkinson's.[2] Even more trivial items like regrowing hair or turning grays back to their normal color and luster might seem impossible, but scientists have discovered that hair follicles harbor stem cells with broad differentiation potential. Researchers are now looking at hair-follicle stem cells for clinical application since they're easy to access compared to the other sources of stem cells.[4] And stem cells are now used to regrow organs such as the liver[5] and even cure many cancers.[6]

The science is still being developed, but who's to say that living comfortably to age 185 will forever be out of the question for the non-yogis among us, even if we don't adhere to a yogi's difficult regimen? The prospects are mind-blowing!

As you embark on this intentional health journey with me and apply the principles of the sages to your modern life, keep your mind open about what your body can do. In truth, the more open-minded you can be, the more your body will be able to do. Let me tell you another quick story that illustrates this fact.

MIND OVER MATTER

Wherever the mind goes, the body will follow. I see this in my practice all the time, such as with my 75-year-old patient Ester. She has a rare blood cancer called *polycythemia vera* that thickens her blood. Periodically, she must have a procedure called a *phlebotomy* to remove blood from her body, which prevents her from developing a blood clot or having a stroke.

Ester has experienced extensive trauma in her life, including two cancers. Despite these challenges, she's a fighter. Her attitude toward life has been instrumental in helping her overcome barriers and beat the odds. She has taught me some valuable lessons too.

She strongly believed, for example, that her body knew how to heal itself. All she had to do was support it. She took a research-supported eight-week mindfulness-based stress-reduction course that helped her change her outlook on her condition even more. Through regular visualizations and meditation, she started feeling much better. She was more attuned to her body and felt empowered in her ability to guide her health intention in a positive direction. After a few months, even her doctors were astonished by her blood results, and she was able to decrease the frequency of her phlebotomy procedures. Mind over matter, indeed.

Separating the mind and spirit from the body is a mistake we've made in Western medicine. As you continue your intentional health journey, always remember the power that your mind and spirit will play in the health of your body.

WALK THIS PATH WITH ME

The first step we'll take on this journey together is to set your individual health intention, which we'll do in Chapter 1. In the subsequent chapters, we'll dive deeper into the ancient health principles of the sages that I use in my practice every day. We'll review the science behind them and discuss real-life examples. You will see how common conditions such as obesity, diabetes, heart disease, and cancer, which are responsible for most of the morbidity and mortality in this country, can be prevented through a unique lifestyle approach that far surpasses just what you eat.[6] Even symptoms such as chronic fatigue, brain fog, irritable bowel syndrome, insomnia, and sluggish metabolism are like flashing engine lights that point to a deeper issue that can be treated. You will learn more about your body from the perspective of both cutting-edge Western and age-old Eastern medicine approaches.

All this knowledge will then be distilled down to a 28-day vitality regimen that you can use to jump-start your journey to optimal health. This regimen helps remove toxins that have accumulated over the years while rejuvenating your organs to function optimally. I know the power of this protocol firsthand, as it enabled me to eliminate debilitating post-COVID-19 symptoms and has helped hundreds of my patients.

The way this book is structured is exactly how I approach every patient in my practice. Through these pages, I invite you into my office so that you can see what truly holistic, patient-centered care looks like. The secret sauce of my trade has nothing to do with me, however. It's all about empowering people to get to know their bodies better and learn how to bring them back into balance.

I know that I might not always be around to help my patients figure out what's going on in their bodies. That's why I equip them with this knowledge, so they can pay closer attention and focus inward to identify imbalances as soon as they occur—before they become diseases. Now you have the benefit of this knowledge too.

Whether you're a young person looking for preventative care, a retired professional seeking longevity and renewed energy, or someone suffering from chronic illness with a rotation of doctors on speed dial, this book will help you become healthier. Once you're armed with its knowledge, you will never look at your body the same way again.

PART I

• • • • • • •

CHARTING THE PATH

CHAPTER 1

YOUR HEALTH INTENTION

The first question I ask all my patients is: *What is your health intention?* They're often surprised by my seemingly simple question, which asks them to envision themselves as healthy. After a pause, they usually say something like, "I don't want to be in pain," or "I don't want my cancer to come back," or "I want to lose weight," or "I don't want to feel tired all the time." It isn't unusual for their response to be accompanied by tears. The one thing I always must have in my office isn't a stethoscope or some fancy medical equipment—it's a box of tissues.

During my years of medical training, I wasn't taught to ask about health intentions. Unfortunately, this approach is far from the norm, so my patients are stunned when I ask what their health means to them. They have never encountered such a question from a doctor, even though it makes perfect sense to initiate our therapeutic relationship with addressing what each individual patient values most.

Unfortunately, most of us spend too much of our lives fearing the worst and praying for something *not* to happen, rather than envisioning our best, healthy selves. When we visualize dreadful scenarios in our heads, we breathe life into them. *That's why setting a positive intention is the most crucial step.* It allows us to channel our healing energy in the right direction.

In order to do that, we have to learn to be intentional with our thoughts. Most of the time, we remain passive participants, simply allowing our brains to carry on with many of the same negative thoughts we've been thinking about ourselves and our lives for years. The brain takes this information from our past experiences, tendencies, and preferences to figure out which thoughts to put forward. It gets out of hand when our mind repeatedly goes to the same scary or punitive places. Often, this leads to uncertainty and anxiety.

Instead, when we're intentional, we become active participants in our thought process. We're in command, instructing our brain where to take our thoughts and which ones to ignore. We set the guidelines about our focus, and our brain obeys these guidelines. It even uses them to channel our subconscious thoughts in the right direction.

When it comes to our health, our thoughts can become either the root cause of a disease or a source of healing. *Whatever we choose to focus on becomes stronger and turns into our reality.* Our attention supercharges our thoughts and intentions. It's like atomic energy stored in a handful of neurons in our brain. This doesn't mean we can control and design every moment of our lives to our specifications, but our health intentions are much more powerful than most people realize.

If you're motivated to change and confident that you can, you can set your intention and direct your brain to think in the way you choose. That's how you become *intentionally healthy.*

POSITIVITY IS YOUR SUPERPOWER

We often think of positive thinking and intentions as merely philosophical, but the process is actually more scientific than that. Think of it as a programming language for your brain. If you want it to work a certain way, you must input the right commands.

Researchers are looking closely now at the intention-related neural response in the brain. There is a widespread distribution of neurons and neural networks for processing our intentions. The findings are helping us figure out how different areas of the brain coordinate with each other to connect our cognition to action.[1]

Our thoughts are dictated by how we feel. If we're having a good day, we tend to have more positive thoughts. The reverse is also true. Research supports the fact that our emotional state can influence our judgments and perceptions of goals. This is why it's important to pay attention to the emotions that dominate our lives.

For example, people with a negative outlook often perceive their health goals to be more difficult compared to their colleagues with a more positive outlook.[2] Of course, no one can feel positive 100 percent of the time, but when we're negative most of the time, it has a significant impact on everything. That's because positivity doesn't just feel good; it has known health benefits. Positive well-being has been associated with nearly a one-third reduction in heart disease in people with high risk factors and as much as a 50 percent reduction in the highest-risk group.[3] That is indeed impressive! Not even blockbuster drugs such as statins or aspirin can promise those kinds of results. Now you see why I call positivity your superpower.

One of the positive emotions that plays an important role in our intentional health journey is *hope*. A greater sense of hope is associated with better physical health and better health behavior outcomes like a reduced risk of all-cause mortality, fewer chronic conditions, a lower risk of cancer, and fewer sleep problems. Hope also provides higher psychological well-being (increased positivity, life satisfaction, and purpose in life), lower psychological distress, and better social well-being.[4] If I could package hope into a pill and give it to everyone, we might not need doctors.

If positivity is so good for us, why does negativity seem to be so much easier? There might be a good reason for that: From an evolutionary perspective, it's advantageous for us to remember our negative experiences so that we can learn from them. Sometimes, negative emotions such as anxiety and fear are necessary to stay vigilant and thwart danger. The tendency to focus on them is often referred to as "negativity bias." It's well researched in the field of psychiatry. Using more of our brainpower to analyze negative emotions and experiences than positive ones is supposed to help us learn faster, giving us an evolutionary advantage.[5]

HOW TO REWIRE YOUR BRAIN

As much as we're hardwired to give more attention to negative thoughts and emotions, we can reprogram our brain to be more positive. There are three things I often encourage my patients to do to shift toward a more positive outlook in life:

1. **Express Gratitude.** I strongly encourage my patients to keep a gratitude journal or start their day expressing gratitude. It has so many physical and psychological benefits. It's also a key ingredient in building resilience. It helps us keep the big picture in mind, so we're less likely to get caught up in trivial matters that trigger a negative reaction. In other words, we don't "sweat the small stuff" as much.

2. **Practice Mindfulness.** Mindfulness is sustained, receptive attention to, and awareness of, events and experiences as they occur. Observing our thoughts helps us to discover what we're thinking mindlessly day in and day out. Often, we're so accustomed to our habitual negative thoughts and emotions that we aren't even aware of them, and we have no idea how much mental energy we're dedicating to them. Mindfulness is about being aware of the present moment. Mindfulness-based exercises have been shown to increase positivity and reduce negativity bias,[6] helping us counteract the negative thoughts that tend to play in our heads on repeat.

3. **Respond Rather Than React.** I call this practice a "stop-and-think moment." Frequently, we find ourselves reacting negatively to certain situations almost as a reflex. Anytime we're stuck in traffic,

someone raises their voice, or our waiter brings us the wrong order, we react with anger, frustration, or fear. On automatic pilot, we bypass the more advanced part of our brain and react using its more primitive part. Usually, the situation doesn't demand such a reaction. Again, this is sweating the small stuff.

Cognitive restructuring is all about taking a pause before we react. This pause gives us an opportunity to analyze our thoughts and decide if a negative reaction is warranted or not. We don't allow the primitive part of our brain to go on automatic pilot. Instead, we choose to respond rather than react. It takes some effort to pause between action and reaction, but it's a skill we can learn. And it's one of the key aspects of cognitive behavioral therapy that I often recommend to my patients. It helps them change how they think and respond more thoughtfully to challenging situations and emotions.

Now that you understand the true power of positivity, let's set *your* health intention.

YOUR HEALTH INTENTION

I believe a question that brings people to tears is a question worth asking, so now, I pose this question to you . . .

What's your health intention?

By asking you to determine your health goals, I'm challenging you to set a positive intention and visualize how you'd like to feel one day. This intention is the first step to healing. Think of it as your "health mission statement."

First, your health intention must be under your control. "I want to live to be 185 years old," or "I want to avoid getting cancer" are tempting options, but they aren't up to us, even as powerful as our thoughts may be. Instead, how about "my health is my priority," or "I'm healing my body by changing how I choose to nourish it"? Those are promises you can make and keep.

Take a moment to close your eyes and envision yourself healthy with lots of energy. What does it feel like? What kinds of things are you doing in your vision that you perhaps can't do now because of a health issue? How does your vision differ from your current day-to-day life? Imagine it as vividly as you can. What do you see, hear, smell, taste, and touch in your mind's eye? Spend some time creating your vision of health. This is where your intention is meant to lead. It's the ultimate desired outcome of your health intention.

Do you have any trouble believing that your vision is possible for you? *It's important that you believe you can achieve your intention.* Setting intentions that you think are unattainable is the Achilles heel for many people. I see patients who are highly motivated to change, but they doubt their ability to do it. This is the litmus test to determine if your intention is within your reach. Just ask yourself the questions, "Can I make this happen?" and "Am I ready to do whatever it takes?"

So, you may need to expand your belief in what's possible for you—but don't discard your original intention *too* quickly. Hold on to it and see if you can magnify your belief by the time you finish reading this book.

Before I send you to the next chapter to read about the wisdom of the sages, I want to say a few words about the concept of karma.

KARMA = ACTION

Most people have heard the word *karma* (which means "action") and even felt the effects of it at times. The Western interpretation of karma is often something like "you reap what you sow" or "tit for tat"—whatever you put in is what you can expect in return. The Eastern interpretation of karma is far deeper than that.

In Hinduism, one of the four spiritual paths is known as *karma yoga*, the path of selfless action. It teaches the spiritual seeker to perform duties without being attached to the outcomes of action. This is indeed a foreign concept to most people. Since the end reward is often what motivates us to perform an action, how can we not be attached to the outcome?

According to karma yoga, attachment is often the root cause of our misery. Regardless of the power of our thoughts and the power of our hope, we can't wholly control our results, so we shouldn't pin our expectations on them. Instead, we should commit to what we *can* control, which is our karma—in other words, *our effort.* As long as we give 100 percent, we have done our part.

I know this is easier said than done. After all, I just asked you to envision yourself healthy! But as you continue through the book, you'll choose specific actions to work toward the *desired* outcome of your health intention. The more you focus on your actions, the easier it will be to maintain your vision without becoming fixated on it. Letting go of attachment is a kind of surrender, trusting that if you do your part, all will work out for your greater good.

Again, action is the key here. Setting the best of intentions but taking no action is like just sitting in a fancy car. It's great to have a nice ride, but a car actually needs to move for us to get closer to our destination. *Our actions put our intentions in motion.* That is how we make progress.

The beauty of intentional health is that we shift to an action-based approach and get into the driver's seat. With this power, we have more control over our health destiny, even as we surrender our attachment to the result.

While addressing only a segment of what karma really is, its Western definition is right about one thing: *what we put in is what we get in return.* The same is true of intentional health.

According to the ancient Indian sages: "You are what your deepest desire is. As is your desire, so is your intention. As is your intention, so is your will. As is your will, so is your deed. As is your deed, so is your destiny."

Now let's turn our attention to the sage wisdom of the ancients and the science that backs up their principles.

PART II

. . . .

SEVEN
ANCIENT
SECRETS

CHAPTER 2

THE CIRCADIAN RHYTHM

Simon was a highly successful CEO who once ran marathons. Then suddenly, he barely had the energy to get out of bed. He went to some of the best doctors and had an extensive blood workup, but he received no real explanation for his fatigue. He was relieved to know he didn't have cancer or another life-threatening condition, but it was terrifying for him to go from high energy to needing ADHD medications and coffee just to get through the day.

I knew the minute I met Simon that what he was experiencing was real and serious. Life-threatening or not, anything that makes you feel unlike yourself and compromises your quality of life must be taken seriously. That's why I had to think outside the conventional medicine box, which had failed to diagnose him even after testing him for virtually everything.

During our first meeting, I reviewed a detailed history, focusing on his diet and lifestyle before his symptoms began. In his 20s and early 30s, he had worked hard to earn success in the business world. Since he dealt with a team distributed across the globe, his typical day started before 5 A.M., and he frequently traveled internationally. All the while, he hit the gym five times a week or more, training for ultramarathons. His life was the epitome of "doing it all."

Unfortunately, success sometimes comes at a high price, putting our body through more than it can handle without time to recover. Eventually, it catches up with us, just like it caught up with Simon. In this chapter, we'll see just how important circadian rhythm is for keeping our body in balance.

THE SCIENCE: CHRONOBIOLOGY

Scientists know that everything in the universe, including us, has a cyclical nature. The tiniest atoms and the largest galaxies are guided by the same fundamental laws. Whether you believe in astrology or not, the planets, sun, and moon directly influence the physiology of every living organism.

The ability to synchronize with natural cycles is the key to evolution and the survival of not only humans but all living creatures. On a crisp fall day, we might not pay much attention to the changing color of the leaves or the squirrels scrambling to stockpile nuts, but everything around us buzzes with activity, all in sync with natural cycles. Bears know to hibernate in winter, trees know when to shed their leaves, and our bodies experience cyclical changes too, even if we aren't consciously aware of them.

We might feel immune to the change of seasons or even the change from day to night, thanks to our light bulbs and thermostats. But our ability to tell night from day and spring from summer has been perfected over millions of years and is vital to our survival. This is why our circadian rhythm, the internal body clock, is in sync with the universe. It guides our different physiological processes over the course of a 24-hour day-and-night cycle, functioning with the accuracy of a Swiss clock.

This internal clock regulates important functions such as our behavior, hormone levels, sleep, body temperature, and metabolism. A disruption of circadian rhythm has been implicated in many conditions from Parkinson's[1] to heart disease,[2] obesity,[3] depression,[4] cancer,[5] and more.

We know all this due to research in a new, multidisciplinary field called *chronobiology*, which is dedicated to studying biological rhythms. In 2017, the Nobel Prize in Physiology or Medicine was awarded to Jeffrey C. Hall, Michael Rosbash, and Michael W. Young for their discoveries of molecular mechanisms controlling the circadian rhythm.[6] Chronobiology has provided valuable insights into how humans, plants, and animals synchronize their biological clocks with Earth's rotation. Current research has just scratched the surface in this field, so expect a lot more in the coming years.

Even though circadian rhythm is in vogue right now in the Western medicine world, our ancestors understood its importance eons ago. Undistracted by television or the Internet, they spent their nights observing the elegant movements of the stars and monitoring other celestial actions to predict changes in their environment. Without this ability, they wouldn't have known when to plant crops or how to prepare for a cold winter. If it hadn't been for the astute observational skills that helped them survive, we might all still be hunter-gatherers.

Eastern medicine has also always recognized the intimate connection between all living creatures and the planets, as well as their cyclical properties. It states that everything in nature, including the body, is made up of five elements: wood, earth, fire, water, and metal. According to traditional Chinese medicine (TCM), each element is associated with a different organ, season, taste, color, and emotion.

Ayurveda has a similar belief that we are made up of five elements, just like everything in nature. It further categorizes different combinations of elements into three *doshas*. Earth and water elements combine to create *kapha dosha*, whereas water and fire create *pitta dosha*, and ether (similar to metal) and air create *vata dosha*. Think of doshas as body types or constitutions. Like our genetic makeup that we inherit from our parents, we also inherit certain dosha tendencies from them.

As we grow up, environmental influences play a bigger role in determining which dosha is more dominant at any given time. Our diet and lifestyle, along with the external environment—such as the climate we live in or the season—also influence our doshas.

Doshas are different from our genes. When we are born, our genetic imprint is given in our DNA, which itself does not change. However, doshas constantly change in response to our behavior and environment. They work as in the science of epigenetics, which focuses on genes being turned on and off. Epigenetics explains why identical twins might have different health destinies. They have the same genetic code; however, which genes are turned on or off entirely depends on their behavior and environment. Similarly, identical twins might have the same DNA, but they have different doshas.

When I see someone for an initial consultation, I often identify which dosha is dominant for them. It helps me understand their physiologic and emotional makeup and how it might have contributed to their condition. Besides identifying the problem, understanding their doshic constitution also helps me come up with a treatment plan that is well suited for them.

For everyone, depending on the time of the day or season, and even their age, one element or dosha might be more dominant than another. Diseases occur when one of the elements becomes too strong or active. Hence, we strive to keep the elements in balance to maintain our health and well-being. Knowing someone's dosha helps me customize a treatment plan to fit them to a *T* (or in this case, to a *D*).

If you're curious, you can take the quiz below and find out which dosha is dominant for you overall, as well as which one might be more prominent currently.

What Is Your Primary Dosha?

Sometimes my patients think that I am a psychic. By looking at their physical features, the way they speak, their general disposition, and even their symptoms, I can determine their primary dosha and which dosha might be causing their symptoms currently. Based on that, I can often predict what their diet, lifestyle, and health issues are.

Trust me, I am no psychic. You might be able to do the same kind of "reading" if you gain some basic understanding of each dosha.

The three doshas are vata, pitta, and kapha. Each has its own unique expression.

Vata is associated with the energy of the wind and motion in our body. It controls our circulation and breathing. When it is in balance, it promotes creativity and vitality. When it is out of balance, it can lead to fear, fatigue, and anxiety.

Pitta is associated with the energy of the fire and our metabolism. It controls our digestion and helps transform food into nutrition. When in balance, it promotes intelligence and contentment. When it is out of balance, it can lead to anger and frustration.

Kapha is associated with the energy of the earth and our strength. It gives structure and cohesiveness to our body and mind. When in balance, it manifests as love and compassion. When it is out of balance, it can lead to inertia and resistance to change.

There are two ways you can take the dosha quiz. First, answer questions based on what has held true for you for most of your adulthood. This will give you a clue to what your dominant dosha is.

Second, retake the quiz and choose answers based on what you have been experiencing over the last few months. The results will give you an insight into which dosha might be overactive or out of balance right now.

Circle each box that applies to you. If more than one characteristic is applicable, you can pick more than one option.

Give yourself one point for each circled box and tally the results. The dosha with the highest number of responses is likely your predominant one. For most people, one is dominant, while others have two doshas—or all three—equally dominant.

However, it's important to note that this is just a general quiz; hence, it may not be entirely accurate. For a more detailed assessment, it's best to consult with a qualified Ayurvedic practitioner.

Dosha Quiz

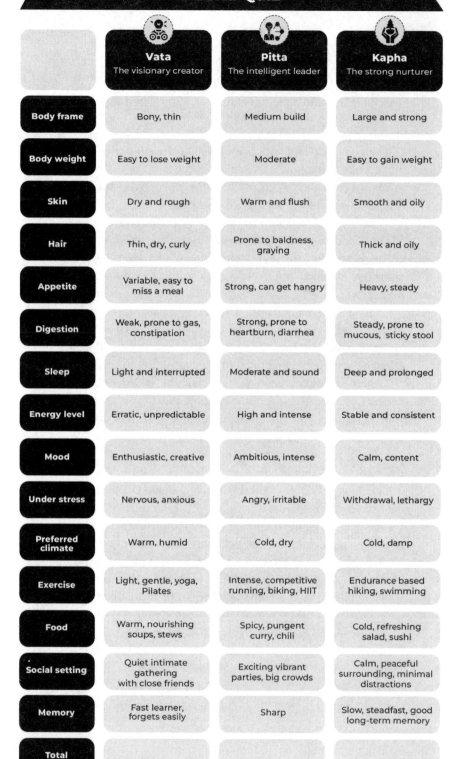

	Vata The visionary creator	**Pitta** The intelligent leader	**Kapha** The strong nurturer
Body frame	Bony, thin	Medium build	Large and strong
Body weight	Easy to lose weight	Moderate	Easy to gain weight
Skin	Dry and rough	Warm and flush	Smooth and oily
Hair	Thin, dry, curly	Prone to baldness, graying	Thick and oily
Appetite	Variable, easy to miss a meal	Strong, can get hangry	Heavy, steady
Digestion	Weak, prone to gas, constipation	Strong, prone to heartburn, diarrhea	Steady, prone to mucous, sticky stool
Sleep	Light and interrupted	Moderate and sound	Deep and prolonged
Energy level	Erratic, unpredictable	High and intense	Stable and consistent
Mood	Enthusiastic, creative	Ambitious, intense	Calm, content
Under stress	Nervous, anxious	Angry, irritable	Withdrawal, lethargy
Preferred climate	Warm, humid	Cold, dry	Cold, damp
Exercise	Light, gentle, yoga, Pilates	Intense, competitive running, biking, HIIT	Endurance based hiking, swimming
Food	Warm, nourishing soups, stews	Spicy, pungent curry, chili	Cold, refreshing salad, sushi
Social setting	Quiet intimate gathering with close friends	Exciting vibrant parties, big crowds	Calm, peaceful surrounding, minimal distractions
Memory	Fast learner, forgets easily	Sharp	Slow, steadfast, good long-term memory
Total			

Now let's look at how different elements and doshas affect our metabolism on a daily basis. In TCM and Ayurveda, the 24-hour clock is divided into segments. Each segment correlates with the element or dosha that's most active at that time. Our ancestors appreciated that our physiology is constantly in motion, changing hour by hour. Physiologically speaking, we aren't the same person at 9 A.M. as we are at 9 P.M.

For example, the large intestine meridian is most active between 5 A.M. and 7 A.M. This is the optimal time to empty our

Traditional Chinese Medicine Clock

Spleen
Convert food into energy
Productivity

Heart
Blood circulation
Lunch

Small Intestine
Absorb nutrients
Nap

Stomach
Digestion
Breakfast

Bladder
Urination
Work, Study

Large Intestine
Bowel movement
Wake up, Exercise

Kidney
Store nutrients
Dinner

Lung
Detox
Dream sleep

Pericardium
Protection
Sex, Self-care

Liver
Detox
Deep sleep

Gall Bladder
Cell repair
Sleep

Triple Burner
Metabolism
Bedtime

Earth · Fire · Water · Metal · Wood · Fire

bowels. If your bowel movements are like clockwork, you can thank your internal clock for keeping you on schedule every morning. If they aren't always on time, your large intestine meridian might need some love.

This clock can also identify imbalances based on which symptoms are happening at a given time. For instance, people with anxiety are more likely to wake up with their mind racing early in the morning, when vata dosha is more active. When out of balance, this dosha often causes anxiety. During menopause, women are more likely to experience hot flashes between 12 A.M. and 2 A.M., which is associated with the liver meridian and pitta dosha, because these can overheat the body.

But don't let these Eastern medicine concepts confuse you. They're simply used in place of Western medicine terms to describe the changes in our physiology hour by hour. While the terminology might be different, the overarching principle is the same. We know for sure, for example, that our body temperature, heart rate, and blood pressure vary depending on the time of day or night. The genes that are activated, the proteins that are made, and the metabolic processes that are turned on and off are all tied to the movement of the sun in the sky.

No wonder that in Eastern medicine, every prescription starts with optimizing the circadian rhythm. *When we synchronize our mealtimes, bedtime, work, and playtime in accordance with our internal clock, our body functions effortlessly. That's the key to preventing diseases and living with vitality.* And that's where Simon ran into trouble.

WHAT GOES WRONG

Even before you're born, you start to synchronize your circadian rhythm with your mother's.[7] As your internal clock keeps track of time, it also communicates with every cell in your body. Without the information, your cells wouldn't know which task to perform. When your rhythm gets out of sync, your cells become confused, which results in significant disruptions in both your body and mind.

We have all had a glimpse of this kind of chaos in the form of jet lag. After a trip across the world, everything from your brain to your bowels is off cycle. But subtler changes in circadian rhythm can also impact our health. Based on Simon's history, I knew his circadian rhythm had taken a beating from his busy work and travel schedule. The early-to-wake-and-late-to-bed routine didn't give his body enough time to recuperate. On top of that, the high-endurance training that had been great for his cardiovascular health at first had started to take a toll. Then, every international trip meant his internal body clock was in a constant state of readjustment.

Any time our circadian rhythm is disrupted, it increases the stress hormone cortisol. Instead of normal fluctuations in cortisol during the day and night, we have a much higher baseline throughout the day. Persistent elevation in cortisol wreaks havoc with our immune system, hormones, metabolism, and sleep. With his lifestyle out of sync with his operating system, everything became an uphill battle for Simon's body.

Let's walk through the three most common symptoms linked to circadian rhythm. It's true that the pathophysiology behind them can be complex and is often multifactorial. However, once you start peeling the onion, you will find the circadian rhythm at the core of it.

Common Symptom #1: Fatigue

No machine can work 24/7, and our body is no exception. In Eastern medicine, health is a balance between yin and yang. In other words, there's a time to work and a time to rest. But sometimes, even if we lie down in bed for 12 hours, we don't feel rested. In that case, how's a tired, cranky person supposed to get through the day?

Fatigue is a sign that our body is working overtime and running out of energy too quickly. It's using up or perhaps wasting a lot of energy doing things it shouldn't have to do. This can happen for several reasons.

First, our bedtime, wake-up time, and mealtimes are often erratic and change every day. The body is a masterful piece of machinery but a creature of habit. Think of it as the most advanced "natural" intelligence system ever created. Artificial intelligence machines learn and get smarter by looking at data and recognizing patterns, which is what our body does naturally. If we go to bed at the same time, wake up at the same time, and have set mealtimes, our body figures out a routine for itself. Half an hour before bedtime, it will start releasing melatonin, getting us ready for sleep. It will also increase acid in the stomach when we're getting ready for lunchtime. It will stay ahead of the game!

If we skip meals, however, sleep at odd hours, and maintain no routine, our body will always have to play catch-up—even as smart as it is. Albert Einstein was such a genius that he could be good at most anything he tried. But imagine asking him to be a doctor one day, a carpenter the next, and a chef another day. Regardless of his exceptional intelligence, he couldn't be an expert at anything by bouncing around professions. On the other hand, a carpenter who has practiced his trade for decades will be able to build a complex cabinet effortlessly, because he's been doing the same thing every day for years. This is also how the human body works. If we allow it to master its trade, it works smoothly in exactly the way it was designed.

We simply can't expect our body to roll with punches every day. Thanks to our modern lifestyle, we frequently try to adapt to new routines, which is exhausting for our body's systems. We might be able to get away with all-nighters in college, whether studying or partying, but we all know that as we get older, we can't bounce back so easily. It starts to add up over time. As we add insult to injury, the disruption in our circadian rhythm becomes the first domino to fall that eventually weakens our immune system,[8] making us more susceptible to illness and more likely to take longer to recover. This also leads to chronic inflammation,[9] which is the root cause of many common conditions like heart disease, arthritis, diabetes, and cancer.

Now you can see how all the biggies in the world of medicine—the circadian rhythm, immune system, and inflammation—are intimately connected. Often, imbalances feed a vicious cycle in which the overworked immune system and rising inflammation in the body drain even more energy and lead to chronic fatigue, which is the number-one complaint I hear about in my office. And my suffering patients have already done lab tests with other doctors to rule out thyroid issues, anemia, and other known causes of fatigue, leaving them with no answers.

I have a different approach. I take fatigue very seriously, because I know it's our body's way of telling us it's out of sync. And fatigue is like a canary in a coal mine that lets us know future diseases need to be prevented. The sooner we can harmonize our rhythm, the better chance we have of staying healthy and living longer.

Common Symptom #2: Sleep Problems

If we could sell sleep, it would be one of the hottest commodities on the market. For someone who struggles with insomnia, a few hours of shut-eye are worth their weight in gold. After fatigue, a lack of good sleep is the second most common complaint I hear of in my office, and often, people have both. Since they're both linked to our circadian rhythm, this is no surprise.

When I try to figure out the root cause of sleep disruption, it can be like a chicken-and-egg situation. Is the fatigue causing sleep issues, or is the lack of sleep causing fatigue? Whichever comes first, however, the root cause is the same.

A normal, healthy circadian rhythm looks something like this: cortisol spikes early in the morning, right before we wake up, to get us ready for the day. Since we haven't had anything to eat or drink during the night, the cortisol helps increase our blood sugar and blood pressure to prevent us from fainting as we get out of bed.

Once we break our fast with *breakfast* and start hydrating, cortisol begins to decrease. With each meal, our cortisol level continues to drop. As bedtime approaches, the level drops below a certain threshold, and this dip activates the release of melatonin to initiate deeper and deeper stages of sleep. A couple of hours before our alarm goes off, the melatonin starts to wind down, making way for cortisol to take over again. These opposing levels of cortisol and melatonin are the foundation of our circadian rhythm.[10]

Unfortunately, the delicate balance is disrupted by our busy, stressful lives. As we start our day with the blaring noise of an alarm, moving on to doom-scrolling on the phone and then off to the races, our stress hormone cortisol starts working overtime right from the get-go. Instead of peaking early in the morning and starting to wind down by midday, it has to remain on duty much longer. As we zoom around all day from meeting to meeting, class to class, or chore to chore, we keep pumping out more stress hormone. By the time evening rolls around, we're still wired from the hormone high. As the wired-and-tired feeling continues, we try to go to bed, but sleep seems elusive. We feel our body about to crash from exhaustion, but we still can't fall asleep because our mind has not slowed down.

The brain may still be thinking about our to-do list and the e-mails we forgot to send. Or we try to unwind and relax by looking at different sizes of screens. Neither of those activities sends the right signal to the brain. With cortisol still lingering in a higher-than-expected range, it prevents the brain from releasing melatonin. To make matters worse, the blue light emanating from the screens tricks our brain into thinking we're still in daytime.

Poor melatonin, nature's sleeping potion, doesn't stand a chance. "There must be a pill for this," we think. Not the addicting, overdosing type, but how about something natural, like a melatonin supplement? I wish popping a few milligrams of melatonin could reset your internal body clock, but it can't. While a supplement might help for a few days, it's no substitute for staying disciplined about how you treat your internal clock during the day, as well as at night.

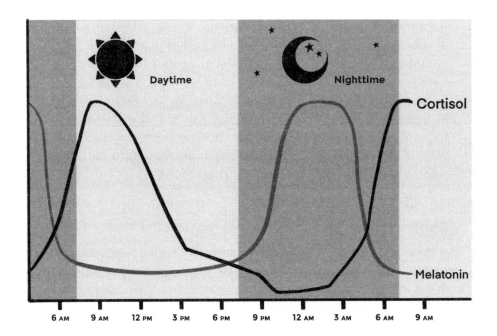

Simply put, if you can't sleep, chances are your stress levels are high throughout the day. Besides stress, irregular mealtimes can prevent the necessary down-trending of your cortisol during the day. *Yes, what you do during the day, including when you eat your meals, has an impact on how well you sleep. Once again, a disciplined routine during the day will lay a foundation for optimal sleep.*

The double whammy of sleep disruption occurs when we add nighttime screen exposure into the mix. Studies have shown that melatonin suppression occurs rapidly—within the first five minutes after we're exposed to bright light[11]—while cortisol levels increase significantly. Even the slightest exposure to blue light has an effect, whether we're partaking of active screen time or just leaving the TV on in the background.

But that's not all. The harmful effects of exposure to artificial light at night go far beyond poor sleep. Research now reveals that routine exposure to artificial light at night—at work, home, and community settings, is linked to increased risk of breast and prostate cancer. To make matters worse, we're also experiencing decreased exposure to natural sunlight during the day, which is critical in resetting our internal clocks and providing us with vitamin D. No wonder the International Agency for Research on Cancer concluded that night-shift work is probably carcinogenic to humans. Lack of light exposure during the day and too much at night is linked to not only cancer risk but also psychiatric, hypertensive, cardiac, and vascular diseases—our so-called "diseases of civilization."[12] Do we need any more reasons to get into a routine and turn down the lights? I don't think so.

Common Symptom #3: The Inability to Lose Weight

If there were a perfect diet or workout plan that led to sustainable weight loss, we wouldn't have to discuss this topic. But here we are. A lot of noise about weight-loss strategies ignores one important fact: *we're all different when it comes to metabolism.* Weight isn't just about calorie intake. If that were the case, two people in the same family eating an identical diet wouldn't be entirely different in terms of weight and health.

Another common mistake is that we tend to look at diet as a means of losing weight, while ignoring the lifestyle component. By "lifestyle," I don't mean exercise; I mean our daily routine. Weight management has less to do with calories than with our hormones such as cortisol, leptin, ghrelin, and insulin.[13] The most important player here is our good old friend cortisol, since it has a direct effect on the rest of our hormones. *This is why I don't simply look at a patient's body mass index (BMI); I also check the levels of these hormones in their body to obtain a clearer picture of metabolic health.*

When I talk to patients about weight loss, I rarely ask them about their diet first. Most people are surprised, since they expect a detailed diet plan from me and a discussion about calories. Instead, I ask them what time they eat their meals, because it's just as important as the content of their meals. Going one step further, I connect the dots between their mealtimes and their bedtime. Through asking them about their daily activities, I can map out their circadian rhythm. Then I can predict what their metabolism is doing at any given time. Even if their diet is perfect, it won't help them lose weight or maintain a healthy weight if it isn't synchronized with their circadian rhythm.

A study published in the *International Journal of Obesity* supports my approach. The findings show that people who eat a higher percentage of their food intake in the morning window instead of the evening have lower odds of becoming overweight or obese. The results were even more startling when they divided the group based on their chronotype—"morning people" versus "night owls." The majority of food intake consumed by night owls at night was associated with approximately a fivefold increase in their odds of being overweight or obese. Also of note is that these associations were stronger for the intake of carbohydrates and protein than for fat.[14]

Most of our food intake, especially carbs and proteins, should be eaten during the day instead of at night. The beneficial effect of this type of diet increases even more when it's tied to a more regular early bedtime and early wake-up time. *Several other studies have validated this concept and demonstrated that breakfast-skipping,[15] late lunch-eating,[16] and high energy intake at dinner[17] have all been linked to weight gain.*

This information isn't meant to simply linger in a research journal. It's time we put it into practice and shift away from the old paradigm of weight loss that's too diet- and calorie-centric.

THE SOLUTION: GET IN SYNC

In almost every patient I see, I can identify at least one symptom or disease that's directly tied to operating out of sync with their circadian rhythm. This is why the first part of any treatment plan I create focuses on establishing a daily routine. It makes sense to synchronize our body first, rather than force it to swim upstream day and night. Any other change to our diet or exercise routine will be far more effective if it goes with the flow.

To test this theory with Simon, I conducted a salivary cortisol test to measure his cortisol levels at different times during a 24-hour period. This helped me map his circadian rhythm. Based on the results, I diagnosed him with adrenal exhaustion.

The adrenal glands are responsible for making cortisol. When they're forced to work overtime, as in Simon's case—pumping out extra cortisol for years—they begin to wear out.

Through a more extensive bloodwork analysis, we also found that Simon had low testosterone levels. This didn't surprise me, because we know the circadian rhythm affects our hormone balance. High levels of cortisol often lead to lower levels of sex hormones like estrogen and testosterone. When we're under high stress, our libido is often the first thing to go.

Fortunately, the rest of his bloodwork was normal. It didn't show any inflammation or autoimmune conditions, which can arise from a chronic disruption of our internal clock. Even before coming to see me, Simon had made some intuitive changes in his lifestyle. Instead of pushing himself so hard, he'd dialed down the intensity of his workouts and added restorative yoga. He'd also made dietary changes and allocated more time for sleep to give his body adequate rest.

At first, he relied on medications and a few cups of coffee to get through the day, but these only caused him to feel more exhausted. So he cut back. Just by listening to his body and aligning his diet and lifestyle accordingly, he began to feel better.

As part of his treatment plan, we worked on diet, sleep, and exercise that would help restore his energy. We also added mind-body practices to build resilience and manage his stress better without burning out. Lucky for him, he was able to move south to warmer weather, which allowed him to spend more time outdoors in nature. There's little like an extra dose of sunshine to reset our clock.

With additional help from herbs and supplements, Simon was able to feel balanced and like himself again within just a few months. His circadian rhythm and his hormones bounced back to normal. He's now working out again in moderation and getting ready to be a dad!

Even if your symptoms are less dramatic than Simon's, it's highly likely that you've suffered from some symptom or other as a result of an out-of-sync internal body clock. And if you haven't so far, I can almost guarantee that you will sooner or later. Here's how I train my patients to resynchronize their circadian rhythm and rebalance their body with intention:

Recognize the Problem

If you suffer from low energy, poor sleep, and/or weight issues, you know something isn't right with your circadian rhythm. Don't ignore it! These symptoms are your body's way of informing you that it's struggling to swim upstream. If you choose to overlook this warning, the problem will only become worse and harder to fix.

Gather Data

Start keeping track of your routines with mealtimes and bedtimes, along with subjective data about how you feel each day and how well you slept. You can use apps, data from your wearable devices, or an old-fashioned journal. If you can also get detailed bloodwork from your doctor, you'll have even more objective measures to monitor.

Patients often think I ask them to track this information just because I want to analyze the data, but it isn't for me. It's to help them gain a deeper insight into what's happening in their body. I won't always be there to tell them what to do, so every person needs to be an expert on their own body. A doctor is merely a guide in the health process. By tracking the data, you'll bring awareness into the process, which will also motivate you to maintain your intention.

Build a Routine

Here comes the hard part—making changes. You know what I'm going to tell you to do: wake up early, avoid skipping meals unless you're truly not hungry, eat a lighter dinner, go to bed at the same time every night, and turn off all screens an hour before bedtime.

I also know what you're probably thinking right now: "I've been a night owl my whole life," or "I'm just not hungry in the morning," or "There's no way I can be in bed by ten." I've heard it all. (Note that there's a caveat to not eating when you aren't hungry: if it's in the morning, eat something even if you don't feel like it. That will stimulate your appetite and begin to reset your rhythm so that you'll be more likely to be hungry at breakfast time.)

If you put in 100 percent effort to synchronize your circadian rhythm, you can expect maximum results. If you try to negotiate your bedtime to midnight, don't be surprised if you get 50 percent of the expected result. If that's okay with you, it's fine by me. But there are no shortcuts when it comes to the most important thing: your health. I'm not making any promises that I haven't been able to fulfill with my patients.

Of course, I'm not saying you can never go out to the theater or take your dream trip to New Zealand. But whenever you veer from your schedule, work hard to get your rhythm back in sync as quickly as possible. And if you have a job like Simon's that requires a lot of international travel, know that it could have a detrimental effect on your health, especially long term.

The Circadian Rhythm/Weight-Loss Solution

When I met my patient Sarah, she had been struggling with weight gain, especially since menopause. She had recently lost her mother to Alzheimer's disease and wanted to do everything she could to optimize her health. We started out with a detailed blood analysis to evaluate her metabolic profile, including inflammation and hormone levels, as well as fasting insulin levels to measure blood sugar.

This kind of detailed blood analysis shifts the focus away from the weighing scale. I do this because I also have patients who fall into the category of "skinny fat." Their BMI might be in the normal range, but other parameters might be abnormal, such as their body-fat percentage, insulin resistance, and levels of hormones such as cortisol and leptin. Ultimately, these are the markers that become the root causes of conditions like diabetes and heart disease.

Next, I got Sarah started on a daily routine for mealtimes and bedtime. We implemented an intermittent fasting window so that she could have her dinner by 7 P.M. and her first meal of the day around 9 A.M. These lifestyle changes increased her energy level and bowel movements. She began losing some weight, and there was a positive change in her blood sugar, cholesterol, and insulin levels.

Sarah was knowledgeable about diet and started exercising regularly as well. She wanted to further personalize her treatment plan, so we added continuous glucose monitoring to gain insight on which foods spiked her blood sugar the most. She also began wearing an Apple Watch and an Oura Ring to track her sleep and heart rate. This gave her real-time data and proof as to how her diet and lifestyle changes were dramatically improving her weight, energy levels, and sleep.

Based on her results and the research mentioned earlier, we changed the macronutrient content of her diet, making lunch the biggest meal with more complex carbs and protein. Her dinner became low carb with more plant-based fat and fiber. This helped keep her fuller longer and reduced her insulin levels.

The knowledge Sarah gained through this process was priceless. She could tell exactly how her body responded to the changes she made. Instead of trial and error, it enabled her to be strategic. This wasn't just about losing a few pounds; it was about bringing her body back to balance with intention.

YOUR PERSONAL ROUTINE

To help you build a routine, I will draw from both Eastern and Western medicine. Eastern medicine places an enormous emphasis on the circadian rhythm. It focuses on maintaining synchronicity by creating a daily and seasonal routine. The following image summarizes the Chinese medicine and Ayurvedic clock concept, highlighting when specific organs and metabolic processes are at their peak. Scheduling your daily routine in coherence with this clock can maximize the benefits from your diet, sleep, and exercise. It can even affect your productivity and ability to focus.

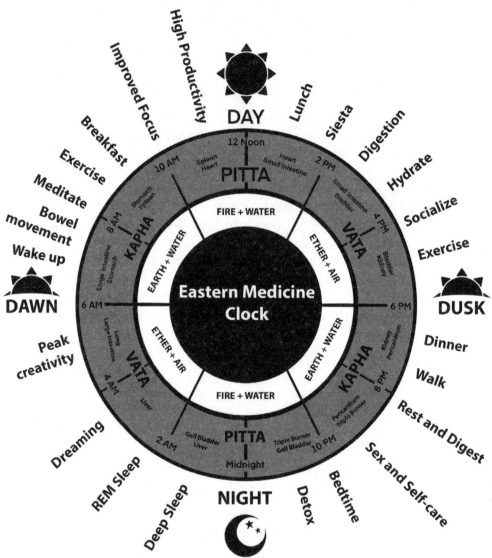

Wake-Up Time

Ideally, you should wake up before the sun rises. This period in Ayurveda correlates with vata dosha, which helps with the elimination of waste from your body. Your large intestine meridian is active then, so it's the perfect time to have a bowel movement—preferably as soon as you wake up.

If you wake up after sunrise or after 8 A.M., you enter the realm of the stomach/spleen meridian, which is related to digestion. This is when your body is ready to break your overnight fast and initiate digestion. Waking up later means skipping the very important elimination step, because you need to empty the colon before you feed the stomach. No wonder constipation is more common in people who wake up later.[18]

For the overachievers and spiritual seekers, the ideal time for creativity and meditation is before sunrise. In ancient Vedic text, the period before sunrise is referred to as *Brahma muhrata*. This period begins one hour and 36 minutes before sunrise and ends 48 minutes before it. Serious yogis wake up before the start of Brahma muhrata, then meditate and do yoga to maximize the benefits of their practice.

As we wake up, our brain is in a theta state of relaxation, which is ideal for the creation of million-dollar ideas.[19] We can enhance our memory[20] and prolong the effect of theta waves through yoga-based practices.

Exercise

The best time to exercise is in the morning.[21] It helps remove stagnation from the body by promoting the elimination of waste and lowering cortisol levels. Studies have shown that a morning exercise routine can improve the quality of your sleep and even lower your blood pressure.[22] As a bonus, you start your day with an extra dose of endorphins. For me, getting exercise out of the way in the morning means I don't have to think about it for the rest of the day. If you really can't make it happen in the morning, another option is in the late afternoon before dinner.

Mealtimes

The ideal time for breakfast is about two hours after waking up. Let's say you wake up at 6:30 A.M., you have a bowel movement and then work out, and by 8:30 A.M., you're ready for some grub. Breakfast doesn't need to be sausage, eggs, bacon, and a stack of pancakes. It should be enough to give you energy until lunch, but not so much that it makes you lethargic. Overeating in the morning will make you reach for an espresso by 10:30 or 11:00, while a lighter breakfast will give you a burst of energy. This is why 10 A.M. to 12 P.M. is considered a great time to organize, plan, and take action. Research shows we're most productive around 11 A.M., and our productivity takes a hit after lunch. So, it's a good idea to get some work done before you get hungry again.[23]

Your digestion is the strongest when the sun is right above your head, which is between 12 noon and 2 P.M. This is the time to eat your largest meal of the day—when your pitta dosha is boosting your digestion and the small intestine meridian is getting ready to absorb nutrients. Based on the research we reviewed earlier, lunch can be more carb-and-protein focused.

After lunch, between 2 and 4 P.M., your energy might be in a bit of a lull. This is why some countries have a siesta at this time. Unfortunately, most of us don't have that luxury, so I recommend scheduling all of your boring meetings during these hours, if possible. From 4 to 6 P.M., you should feel another burst of energy, because this is after your lunch has been digested. If you didn't work out in the morning, this is a good time to squeeze it in. It's also an ideal time to socialize, according to Ayurveda. (Did someone say "happy hour"?)

A workout and socializing might whet your appetite and get you ready for dinner, which is ideally before sunset. The last thing our ancestors wanted to do was wander around in the dark eating a meal, since they were more likely to *become* a meal at that time. On average, it takes three hours for our food to be digested and leave the stomach. If we eat dinner by 7 P.M., there's ample time for the body to digest before bedtime. It isn't ideal to go to bed with food in the stomach. For these reasons, we evolved to eat an earlier, lighter dinner.

By following this mealtime schedule, you're automatically fasting for 12 to 14 hours every night. Intermittent fasting might be all the rage right now, but it was simply part of life for our ancestors. Another major benefit of this overnight fasting window is that it helps reduce cortisol and improve insulin sensitivity. Both of those play a key role in our metabolism and weight.[24]

One of the barriers to eating an earlier dinner is that we get hungry later at night, especially if we're used to going to bed late. The closer we get to midnight, the more likely we are to see a spike in cortisol if we aren't fast asleep. This makes us hungry and prevents melatonin secretion. *I recommend eating a lighter dinner that has fewer carbs and proteins with healthy, plant-based fats and a lot of fiber to keep you fuller longer. I generally like to avoid carbs at night, since they're more likely to send insulin and cortisol levels on a roller coaster.* Then you won't crave ice cream or desserts as you watch TV and unwind. A lower-carb dinner keeps your insulin levels low through the night, which also help you burn fat.[25]

I love my carbs in all shapes and forms, but I make a point to eat most of them during lunch instead of dinner. If I want to enjoy pizza or pasta, I prefer eating them during the day. If I do eat them for dinner, I keep the portion sizes small and eat more fiber (extra veggies for the pizza topping) and protein (a side of lentil soup) with them. There are some days when my appetite is low, and I don't feel like eating a big dinner. When I'm not that hungry in the evening, I opt for an herbal tea instead.

Bedtime

After a long day of work, who doesn't look forward to unwinding with a glass of wine or a good TV show to go along with a bowl of ice cream? It's so easy to lose track of time when there's an endless buffet of entertainment at your fingertips. Gen Z might not be used to it, but back in the day, we had to wait a whole week to watch a new episode of our favorite show, only to have it constantly interrupted by commercials. I would be lying if I said I missed those interruptions, but in a way, they served a purpose. They provided a break so we could come back to reality and do a time check. Today, most of us are so used to scrolling through social media or spending hours browsing through streaming services that it's time for bed before we know it—or we miss that ideal bedtime window entirely.

Remember that bedtime is a lot more than just hitting the sack. Our body goes through that cortisol-to-melatonin transition and from digestion to detox, both of which are critical for our health. Any mixed signals during this time will have a significant impact.

Unlike us, our ancestors didn't have to worry about the light-pollution exposure of urban environments. For us, it's a constant problem that disrupts our pineal gland, preventing it from releasing enough natural melatonin at the right time and in the right amount. In our modern world, we're hard-pressed to find true darkness. Research has shown that an increased amount of light at night lowers melatonin production, which results in sleep deprivation, fatigue, headaches, stress, anxiety, and other health problems. And blue light is the worst.[26]

Unfortunately, besides our TVs, tablets, and cell phones, blue light is also emitted from energy-efficient LED lightbulbs. We just can't seem to get away from it. Imagine watching TV into the evening and then trying to go to sleep. Your pineal gland hasn't had a chance to make the switch to night mode yet. Even if you do fall asleep, it might be a while before you enter the deep-sleep stage. Studies have found that the ratio of deep sleep significantly decreased in groups exposed to blue light compared to groups exposed to incandescent light and using blue-light-blocking glasses.[27] This might explain why even after eight hours of sleep, we might not wake up fully rested and recharged.

Before I knew of this research, I didn't think a little bit of light exposure would make much of a difference. As an avid fan of horror movies, I often slept with the TV on at night to ward off the "boogeyman." But when I discovered the potential link between blue-light exposure and obesity and cancer, I knew I had to change my habit.

A team led by Dr. Dale Sandler at the National Institute of Environmental Health Sciences used data from more than 43,000 women aged 35 to 74 years to study the impact of night-light exposure and weight over a period of about five and a half years. The women were asked whether they slept with no light, a small night-light, a light outside of the room, or a light or television on in the room. The researchers found that women who slept with a light or television on were more likely to be obese at the beginning of the study. They were also 17 percent more likely to have gained about 11 pounds or more over the follow-up period. However, a small night-light wasn't associated with any more weight gain than sleeping with no light, and the association with light coming from outside of the room was more modest.[28]

In my opinion, blue-light exposure through screen time is one of the most ignored culprits that disrupts our circadian rhythm. Therefore, when I see patients with fatigue, insomnia, or weight issues, I pay particular attention to it. A few simple steps, such as avoiding screens a couple of hours before bedtime, wearing blue-light-blocking glasses in the evening, and adjusting the setting on your phone to night mode after sunset can make a big difference.[29] And when you go to bed, I encourage you to use blackout curtains and motion-sensor yellow night-lights, and to turn off all electronics.

Once the blue light is blocked, focus on your actual bedtime. The ideal time to go to bed is between 10 and 11 P.M. For the night owls out there, this might seem like an impossible task. But let me try to scare you into going to bed early. Night owls are 30 percent more likely to have high blood pressure and two and a half times more likely to be diabetic![30] They also tend to consume 248 more calories a day, twice as much fast food, and half as many fruits and vegetables as those with earlier sleep times.[31] If that isn't enough, a large-scale study in the United Kingdom evaluated more than half a million people and found that night owls had a 10 percent higher risk of dying over the six-and-a-half-year study period.[32] That's what I call a true nightmare!

As scary as these statistics are, the silver lining is that focusing on your routine to get your circadian rhythms in sync is a lot easier than dealing with an invasive surgery or chronic illness. It's all about working smarter, not harder.

TIPS FOR OPTIMIZING YOUR CIRCADIAN RHYTHM

Create a schedule for each day. This is the most important commitment you can make on your journey toward intentional health. As part of their homework, I give my patients the following template and ask them to fill it out with times that work for them and post it on their refrigerators:

- *Wake-up time:* The best time to wake up is before sunrise. An hour before sunrise is the ideal time for a meditation practice.

- *Exercise:* The ideal time to exercise is in the morning or late afternoon.

- *Breakfast:* Wait an hour or two after you wake up to eat breakfast.

- *Lunch:* This is your biggest meal of the day. Feel free to enjoy complex carbs and a protein of your choice.

- *Dinner:* The last meal of the day should be around sunset or before. Avoid simple carbs and eat more plant-based fats and fiber to keep your hunger satisfied through the night.

- *Bedtime:* Allow three to four hours between your last meal and bedtime.

If you stick to this routine, you'll be well on your way to resetting your circadian rhythm and achieving the improved health that accompanies it.

CHAPTER 3

THE GOOD BACTERIA

The first time I meet a patient, the questions I ask often catch them off guard. They aren't the kinds of questions most doctors ask. One question in particular makes them blush. No, I'm not talking about their sex life, although I also ask about that. I'll give you a clue: the question contains a word that would have made you giggle when you were a child.

It's poop.

I've been surprised to discover that it's easier to talk about sex than poop. But I'm not one to shy away from asking about the shape, color, smell, and texture of the business that takes place in the bathroom. Since I don't have X-ray vision, the next best thing is to ask about what patients put in their body via their diet and what comes out the other end. In Ayurveda, they say you can tell everything about a person's physical health by asking about their poop and digestion.

In this chapter, I want to focus on our digestive health, and that means a candid discussion of the gut. If the body were a machine, the gut would certainly be the engine, since it's responsible for taking in fuel in the form of food and converting it into energy. But where exactly is the gut? If I asked my two-year-old niece that question, she'd likely point to her belly button. But little does she know that an adult gut is more than 20 feet long! It starts at the mouth and includes the tongue, food pipe, stomach, small and large intestines, rectum, and anus. The gut is a long tube, and each section has its own unique form and function.

In Eastern medicine, the gut is essentially considered the center of the body's universe. The belief is that every disease starts in the gut, so treatment of every disease also starts there. Western medicine is finally starting to catch up with this concept, given the amount of research focusing on the gut microbiome.

The microbiome consists of the trillions of bacteria and other microorganisms in the gut. We now know that these little critters play a crucial role in modulating almost every function in the body from our immune system to our hormones to even neurotransmitters.[1] More than 80 percent of neurotransmitters and "happy" hormones like serotonin and dopamine are made in the gut, not the brain. Clearly, the gut demands more respect than the label "poop factory."

Our gut is intimately connected to our circadian rhythm. What time we eat, how long we take to digest our food, and how and when we eliminate send signals to the brain. These signals in turn help the brain keep track of time and synchronize itself with our master clock. Since we eat several times a day and ideally poop once or twice a day, there is constant communication along the gut-brain axis. Recent evidence indicates that the gut microbiome and circadian genes can interact with each other.[2] That's why our gut health is one of the most important factors in keeping our master clock in sync. Not only that, disruption of the circadian system in turn can alter microbiome communities and perturb our metabolism, energy balance, and inflammatory pathways, which can lead to diseases.[3]

That's why I make a big deal out of gut health. I almost sound like a broken record when I talk to my patients about the root cause of their ailments. If they come to me for depression, I say it's the gut. If they come to me for obesity, I say it's the gut. If they want to stop hair loss, I say it's the gut. Of course, if they want to figure out why they're always bloated and gassy, I say it's the gut.

If I were evaluating patients solely from the perspective of Western medicine, I would send them to a psychiatrist for depression, an endocrinologist or a weight-loss surgeon for obesity, a dermatologist for hair loss, and a gastroenterologist for irritable bowel syndrome. However, when I don my Eastern medicine hat, I start peeling the layers of the onion to figure out how I can address the root cause of these seemingly unrelated symptoms. To achieve optimal health, prevent disease, and treat disease, it's wise to understand the inner workings of this important organ system called the microbiome, and its trillions of residents.

THE SCIENCE: THE MICROBIOME

As humans, we take pride in being the most intelligent and complex organism on the planet. We may not have been around for that long, but from an evolutionary perspective, we've come far in what seems like the blink of an eye.

We may not have a cheetah's speed, an elephant's strength, or a dog's powerful sense of smell, but through ingenuity and innovation, we can now be the fastest, strongest, and smartest. Here we are, walking around with our smartphones, while the chickens and fish are still doing what they've done for millions of years. What gives us this unique advantage?

When DNA was discovered in the 1950s, we thought we'd found the holy grail of our existence. Our genome, which is made up of all the genes that contain our DNA, is like the black box of an airplane. All we had to do was decode the genome to unlock the secret to all our health problems—or so we believed. We were sure we'd cure everything from baldness to cancer. Why even wait to get diseases? Why not check all the genes in a human embryo and correct the imperfections before someone is even born?

Yet, more than 70 years after DNA was discovered and 20 years after the genome was decoded, people are still fighting receding hairlines and cancer. It turns out that our genes are a bit more complicated than we thought. Our idea of linking one gene to one disease didn't pan out. In fact, it was a shocking revelation when we started to decode the genomes of other organisms.

Take a moment to guess the number of genes in a grape, a chicken, a fruit fly, and a human. You would think a human has the most genes. After all, we, not chickens, are the ones with airplanes and the Internet. But a grape has more genes than a human being, while chickens and fruit flies aren't far behind us. On the other hand, a flu virus has only 11 genes, but as anyone who has ever had the flu can attest, those 11 genes can wreak some havoc.

We'd like to believe that humans are the most complex organisms, but we don't have enough genes to claim the top spot in that chain. Instead, we've managed to find another way by making a deal with trillions of tiny bacteria. In exchange for food and shelter, this army of microbes has let us borrow their genetic machinery.

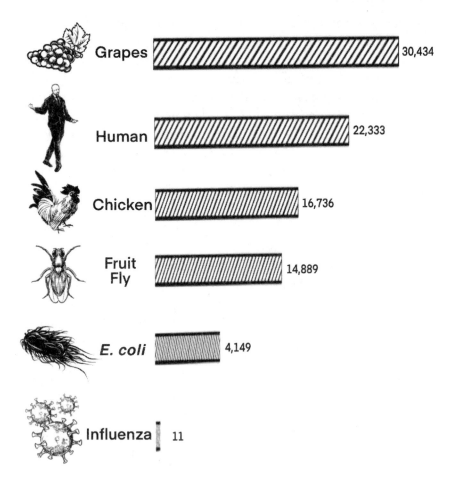

	Genes
Grapes	30,434
Human	22,333
Chicken	16,736
Fruit Fly	14,889
E. coli	4,149
Influenza	11

We have 10 times more microbial cells than human cells in our body. How's that for an identity crisis? But when we combine our 22,000 genes with about a thousand different types of microbes, we have access to more than 3 million genes!

Often, it's the tiny bacteria in and on our body that run the show. After being on the planet for billions of years, they've mastered the art of survival by adapting to their environment. There's no place in the world where you won't find these little guys. They're in the hottest geothermal springs and the coldest parts of Antarctica. They can even survive in outer space. Let's talk about how these bacteria play a role in health and disease.

First, I want to define the term *human microbiome* more thoroughly. It refers to the collective genomes of the microbes that live inside and on the human body, such as bacteria, fungi, protozoa, and viruses. They can be found on our skin and in the mouth, as well as in our gut and vaginal canal. The highest concentration of these bacteria is found in the gut, which is why the term *gut microbiome* has taken center stage in cutting-edge research. To study the human as a "supraorganism" composed of both nonhuman and human cells, the National Institutes of Health (NIH) launched the Human Microbiome Project in 2007 as an extension of the Human Genome Project.

Thanks to the recent interest in studying the gut microbiome, we've learned a tremendous amount. Most health conditions we see nowadays are associated with a disruption of the bacteria balance in the gut. These include diabetes,[4] obesity,[5] heart disease,[6] inflammatory bowel disease (IBD),[7] Crohn's disease, celiac disease,[8] eczema,[9] psoriasis, arthritis,[10] Alzheimer's disease, Parkinson's disease, multiple sclerosis,[11] autism, depression, anxiety,[12] and more. Having thousands of research studies supporting these findings is great, but how can we put this knowledge into practice?

Welcome back into my office. We now know about the role of the microbiome in the functioning of our immune system, hormones, and neurotransmitters. We can bring the latest science to life by marrying technology with the age-old wisdom of Eastern medicine.

WHAT GOES WRONG?

What goes wrong with this microscopic ecosystem in our body? Our gut houses 70 percent of our immune system. This location makes sense, since we're exposed to foreign substances through food three or more times a day.[13] Food can bring in uninvited guests like pathogenic bacteria, viruses, and parasites. If we don't have a very strong gut immune system, eating a bad piece of chicken with a dash of *E. coli* can kill us.

The gut immune system works overtime and is hypervigilant, acting quickly if a threat is identified. It also plays an important role in creating a gut-blood barrier. Think of this barrier as a defense wall that prevents the nasty bugs in the gut from going all over the body and spreading infection. One of the main keepers of this wall and the gut immune system is the gut microbiome. With an army of trillions of bacteria, we can keep enemies at bay.

Just like our military has the army, navy, and air force, our immune system has different branches that specialize in killing certain types of pathogenic bacteria. Our "armed forces" comprise a highly intelligent system that trains itself and learns throughout our life.

But when something disrupts our "armed forces," our gut microbiome gets out of balance. We end up with too many harmful bacteria and too few good bacteria. The following are three common symptoms or conditions caused by issues with the gut microbiome.

Common Symptom/Condition #1: Food Allergies

Whether you avoid gluten because you suffer from celiac disease or no longer eat dairy products because you're lactose intolerant, it's because we live in an era where certain foods have become our enemies. The discomfort they cause can range from unpleasant flatulence to anaphylactic shock. Since we must eat food to survive, living with food allergies can be like walking in a minefield. While some people may have been able to identify their personal kryptonite, others struggle to figure out which foods make them sick.

How exactly do innocent foods like peanuts become so deadly for some people?

As I mentioned, from the day we're born, our immune system continuously evolves based on our individual experiences and exposures. The more encounters we have with bacteria, viruses, and parasites early in life, the better our immune system is trained. If we grow up in a more sterile and "clean" environment, our immune system has fewer opportunities to learn and grow smarter.

When I grew up in India, food allergies were unheard of. Peanuts were never banned from schools, and my classmates didn't have to carry an EpiPen. What was common in India at that time was catching a plethora of bacterial and parasitic infections at a young age. Our immune systems received many important lessons early in life to know that they didn't need to overreact to foods like peanuts or gluten. This idea, called the "hygiene hypothesis," suggests that lack of exposure to parasites in childhood makes the immune system more likely to overreact when it encounters benign allergens.[14]

Understanding how these changes in our microbiome lead to diseases is revolutionizing the development of unique treatments for food allergies. Since we've figured out that allergies are often caused by a disruption in the gut microbiome, the theory is that we could treat them by adding more diverse bacteria. Researchers in Australia treated children with severe peanut allergies with a combination of probiotics and pills that contained small doses of peanut protein. Within a month, these kids showed reduced reactivity to peanuts. When the researchers followed up with the participants, they found out that even after four years, the effects of the treatment persisted.[15]

When we talk about food allergies, we often think about kids. However, in my practice with adult patients, such allergies are still a big issue. Recent studies have found that more than 10 percent of U.S. adults are food allergic, while nearly 19 percent of adults believe they have a food allergy.[16] Even if someone didn't suffer from allergies as a child, they aren't immune to them as an adult.

Many adverse food reactions can have a significant impact on health and quality of life, causing fatigue, pain, and other health issues.[17] Besides physically, they can affect us emotionally and socially. Simple decisions like what to eat for lunch can become tedious and difficult on a daily basis.

I also see the impact of hidden food allergies on overall health. They might not cause anaphylaxis, but they can worsen other conditions, such as migraines,[18] chronic fatigue,[19] and weight gain. For this reason, I often incorporate a detailed food allergy blood test as part of my assessment. For example, I order the food sensitivity test for almost all patients who suffer from chronic migraines. This test analyzes more than 170 types of foods and chemicals toward which we might develop a sensitivity.[20] Every time we ingest that food or become exposed to those chemicals, our immune system gets activated. This can lead to symptoms like a migraine attack. Using food sensitivity testing, I'm able to create customizable dietary recommendations that can help treat migraine headaches, sometimes even without the use of medications.[21] For patients already on medications, it still makes sense to consider this approach for migraines and many other symptoms.

Common Symptom/Condition #2: Autoimmune Diseases

Gut bacteria do an amazing job at helping our immune system differentiate between friends and foes. And since our immune system is used to having bacteria in the gut, it doesn't sound off any alarms when it sees friendly, familiar faces. But if it can't tell the difference between which bacteria are good for us and which are going to make us sick, it remains constantly on its toes, rapid-firing at anything that comes its way.[22]

When our immune system isn't very experienced and doesn't have a diverse army of good bacteria, it gets activated too often, too easily. When it goes into unwarranted action too frequently, we're likely to develop an autoimmune disease such as Crohn's disease, lupus, rheumatoid arthritis, or psoriasis. Then the immune system begins to damage our normal cells without enough time for the cells to repair.[23]

In developed countries where our gut microbiomes aren't as diverse, we see much higher incidences of autoimmune conditions. Frequent antibiotic use is one of the reasons, because it's associated with a higher risk of autoimmune conditions. Antibiotics wipe out many good bacteria in the gut, which are our first line of defense. Studies have shown that even a few rounds of antibiotics early in childhood can significantly increase the risk of autoimmune disease later in life.[24] Therefore, if we want a strong immune system, we need a diverse army of microbes in our gut.

Just a few decades ago, autoimmune conditions weren't that common. Unfortunately, young people are bearing the brunt of this phenomenon. According to the National Institutes of Health, children aged 12 to 19 had a threefold increase in autoimmune markers over the last three decades—the largest increase of any group. Clearly, our genes didn't change in such a short period of time. Other factors must be responsible, including diet, exposure to antibiotics, and/or environmental toxins.[25]

One of the autoimmune conditions I often see in my practice is inflammatory bowel disease, which includes Crohn's disease and ulcerative colitis. This condition is caused by chronic inflammation in the gut, leading to pain, bleeding, and bowel obstruction, sometimes even necessitating surgical removal of the bowels.

When I attended medical school (in this same century, by the way), I learned that this condition is most common among adults in their 50s, but that isn't what I see in my practice now. It's heartbreaking to see teenagers and young adults with their whole lives ahead of them coping with this serious chronic illness.

According to the Centers for Disease Control and Prevention (CDC),[26] about three million adults currently live with inflammatory bowel disease. That's a significant increase compared to two million in 1999. There are newer drugs on the market that are showing promising results. They block part of the immune system to reduce gut inflammation—but this can have many side effects. We don't have long-term studies yet to evaluate the safety profile of these medications. When we treat people in their teens and early 20s with these heavy-duty medications, we even have to consider long-term side effects.

Common Symptom/Condition #3: Breast Cancer

As a woman and someone who has several family members with breast cancer, it's something I worry about, and I have a valid reason to be concerned. The rate of increase in female breast cancer has been more than fourfold since the 1970s, compared to the increase in the U.S. population during that same period. It has outpaced the rise of other cancers such as colon, lung, and uterine.[27] With one in eight women expected to get the disease,[28] we need to ask why.

When we talk about breast cancer, the major player in the story is estrogen, since 70 percent of breast cancers are "estrogen receptor-positive subtype." The cancer cells carry estrogen receptors on them, and the higher the amount of estrogen circulating in the body, the faster the cancer cells grow.

What always perplexed me, however, is that most women are diagnosed with breast cancer after menopause. By that time, the estrogen levels have reduced significantly. So why are cancer cells growing more after menopause, and where is the extra estrogen coming from?

Enter the gut microbiome. "Garbage disposal" is one of the many jobs done by the busy bacteria in the gut. They're responsible for working with the liver to eliminate extra estrogen in the body. If we don't have friendly garbagemen in the gut, however, it can all go very wrong.

Many bad bacteria in the gut produce an enzyme called *beta-glucuronidase*. Instead of deactivating estrogen, this enzyme activates it and sends it back into our blood, where we end up reabsorbing rather than releasing it. The excess hormone circulating in the body can cause polycystic ovary disease, endometriosis, infertility, and even cancers of the breast, uterus, ovary, and prostate.[29]

Until now, we've had limited options to treat conditions like polycystic ovary disease and endometriosis. The usual options included hormonal birth control, which some women can't tolerate. To prevent breast cancer, we recommended regular mammograms, but that was about it.

Today, we have the option to measure beta-glucuronidase levels in the stool, along with profiling the bacteria in the gut and treating related conditions at the root cause. Identifying imbalances early might prevent hormone-related cancers as well. Therefore, diet, exercise, stress management, and reducing exposure to environmental toxins are all important for cancer prevention. They all work by creating a healthy microbial environment in the gut.

Especially for women with a history of breast cancer, it makes sense to check beta-glucuronidase levels in the stool. It can help us customize diet and probiotic recommendations to reduce their risk of developing breast cancer. Studies have shown, for example, that the level of this enzyme is significantly higher in the stools of subjects on a high-meat diet as compared to a non-meat regimen.[30] So, a plant-based diet is often part of the prescription for women with estrogen imbalance.

Gut Bacteria and Testosterone

Women aren't the only ones affected by gut imbalances, of course. As we see an increase in hormone-related conditions in women, there's a similar trend in men. Testosterone levels in men are equally influenced by the bacteria in the gut. Low testosterone is becoming more and more common, and we're diagnosing it at an earlier age than in the past. There are many factors responsible for testosterone decline, including age, exposure to environmental toxins, medications, diet, lack of exercise, and stress. But the good news is that researchers have found that supplementation with *Lactobacillus reuteri* bacteria in mice reduced inflammation and restored testosterone to youthful levels in older mice.[31] Perhaps the fountain of youth is the milieu of bacteria hiding in our gut.

THE SOLUTION: STRENGTHEN
AND PROTECT THE MICROBIOME

When I met my patient Yani, he was experiencing significant symptoms from ulcerative colitis. He sometimes had as many as 15 bloody bowel movements a day with severe abdominal pain. He even had to be admitted to the hospital and treated with IV medications.

When he came to my office, his symptoms were manageable with medications, but he still had frequent flare-ups, which caused him discomfort and required him to take time off from work.

Through a detailed stool microbiome test, we were able to identify what was really going on in Yani's gut. We found two harmful bacteria that are resistant to treatment, along with a significant scarcity of the good guys. Other biomarkers in the stool pointed to a less-than-ideal environment for gut healing with very low levels of butyrate, which is used as fuel for the gut cells to repair themselves. Low levels of butyrate are associated with worsening inflammation in IBD patients and a poor response to treatment.[32]

We combined gut microbiome testing and food sensitivity analysis to come up with a customized diet for Yani. We used other herbs, supplements, and probiotics to slowly shift the balance toward favorable bacteria and gut healing. We even added medical marijuana to his regimen to help with pain and curb inflammation.[33] Acupuncture was very helpful for him too. In several clinical trials, gut microbial composition came closer to normal and the levels of inflammatory molecules were significantly reduced in patients who had acupuncture treatment, which also stimulates intestinal healing.[34] I can't think of a better example of cutting-edge Western medicine and Eastern medicine coming together.

After a few months, Yani felt much better with fewer and less severe flare-ups. He was able to stop most medications, and his most recent colonoscopy was almost normal, with hardly any signs of inflammation. His blood tests also normalized. It's encouraging to know we can put the latest research into practice to optimize gut health.

By using advanced microbiome testing and addressing the root cause, I've been able to treat a multitude of symptoms and diseases while preventing other ailments. We're already in an era where a stool test gives us just as much information, if not more, than a blood test.

Still, a lot of people spend a fortune on probiotic foods and supplements, hoping it will buy them a healthy gut microbiome and not realizing it isn't that simple. Most patients I see in my practice eat a healthy diet and take probiotic supplements. Despite these measures, some of them still suffer from imbalances. That's because we're exposed daily to several hidden threats to our microbiome. We must first avoid these dangers so we can get the most out of our efforts. Let's examine each of these culprits.

Rein In the Antibiotics

While antibiotics can be lifesaving when truly warranted, we must try our best to avoid taking them. As I mentioned before, even a few rounds of antibiotics early in life can lead to several gastrointestinal, immunologic, and neurocognitive conditions.[35] Our gut doesn't just snap back to normal. Unfortunately, according to the CDC, about a third of antibiotics prescriptions in the U.S. are unnecessary,[36] and their rampant use breeds resistance. As a result, infections become harder and harder to treat, because we become immune to the antibiotics we have available. Eventually, we might even run out of treatment options. No wonder the World Health Organization considers antibiotic resistance to be one of the biggest threats to global health, food security, and development.

If you have an infection, it's important to get in the habit of asking your health-care provider for tests that can narrow down the pathogen that's causing it. This can help your doctor pick the most effective antibiotic and for the right duration. Broad-spectrum antibiotics cast a much wider net and can affect many different types of bacteria; they kill the good bacteria in your gut as well as the bad. Testing might even eliminate the consideration of antibiotics altogether if the illness is caused by a virus, which is often the case. Antibiotics simply don't work against viruses.

If you do have to take antibiotics, make sure you complete the prescribed course, even if you start feeling better after a few days. That's another way to prevent resistance.

To protect your gut microbiome during this time, pay extra attention to your diet. A plant-based diet that's high in probiotic-rich foods can help. You should also take a probiotic for the duration of the antibiotic treatment and for several weeks afterward.[37] When taking antibiotics and probiotics simultaneously, however, separate them by a few hours. Theoretically, the antibiotic can neutralize the probiotic if you take them at the same time.

Minimize Pesticides

Next on the list of things to avoid are pesticides. I put them in the same category as antibiotics, since they're meant to kill pests just like antibiotics are meant to kill infection-causing bacteria. Pesticides have been found to have a similar negative impact on the gut microbiome.[38] Besides that, long-term exposure is often associated with diseases like cancer, hormonal disorders, asthma, and allergies.[39]

Buying organic produce is one of the steps you can take to minimize pesticide exposure. Organic doesn't mean zero pesticides, but it generally means fewer than in nonorganic fruits and vegetables. If you're concerned about cost, you don't have to buy everything organic. I always refer to the Dirty Dozen™ list published by the Environmental Working Group (EWG) for which fruits and veggies have the highest amount of pesticide residue.[40] Their Clean Fifteen™ list tells you which produce you can safely buy nonorganic. Fruits and vegetables on that list usually have a peel or thick skin that you remove prior to eating, which minimizes your exposure. Each year, the EWG updates the lists. For example, here are the lists for 2023:

👍 EWG Dirty Dozen™ (Buy organic)	👎 EWG Clean Fifteen™ (No need to buy organic)
Strawberries	Avocados
Spinach	Sweet corn
Kale, collard greens, and mustard greens	Pineapples
	Onions
Peaches	Papayas
Pears	Sweet peas (frozen)
Nectarines	Asparagus
Apples	Honeydew melon
Grapes	Kiwi
Bell peppers	Cabbage
Cherries	Mushrooms
Blueberries	Mangoes
Green beans	Sweet potatoes
	Watermelon
	Carrots

Besides apples, which are usually on the hit list of the Dirty Dozen every year, there are two other things on my grocery list that I *always* buy organic: soy- and oat-based products. Most of the soy produced in this country is meant to feed animals, not humans. Norwegian scientists published a new study showing that high levels of glyphosate—the active weed-killing chemical in the herbicide Roundup—are found in GMO soy. Organic soy doesn't contain as many pesticides, and it's nutritionally superior to GMO soy.[41] So, spend the extra couple of bucks on organic tofu, soy milk, and edamame the next time you shop.

As for oats, pesticides like glyphosate are used to not only kill pests on the crop but also as a desiccant to dry it out. This allows for an earlier harvest and improves crop uniformity.

According to researchers, glyphosate is found in much higher levels in oats because of this practice.[42] No wonder a recent EWG study found more glyphosate than some vitamins in samples of oat-based breakfast cereals marketed to children. For example, in General Mills's Honey Nut Cheerios, the amount of glyphosate exceeded the amount of both vitamin D and vitamin B_{12}. In a sample of Quaker Oatmeal Squares, there was more glyphosate than vitamin A.[43] These are the foods we think are good for our kids, especially if we're trying to avoid gluten and dairy. Oat milk and steel-cut oats are staples in any supposedly healthy kitchen pantry. Now that you have this information, always buy organic oat products.

Whether you buy organic or not, however, you must wash your fruits and veggies thoroughly before you eat them. Take apples, for example. Most of them in grocery stores have been washed in a bleach solution to get rid of bacteria. Now imagine just rinsing one without scrubbing and taking a bite.

A study conducted by researchers at the University of Massachusetts, Amherst, found that soaking apples in a solution of baking soda and water for about 15 minutes helps to remove pesticide residue. This method won't remove all pesticides, since some do penetrate the fruit,[44] but it's better than eating apples dipped in bleach. I personally soak all produce in warm water with baking soda for 15 minutes and rinse it thoroughly before eating. You can also get in this habit with all your produce before you put it away, having it ready to eat whenever you like. I use the ratio of one teaspoon of baking soda to two cups of water. You can also use a vinegar and water solution, but I'm not a fan of the smell or the taste of it on my produce.

I will also take this opportunity to give a shout-out to local farmers' markets. Common sense dictates that if you buy blueberries in the summer, they're likely coming from a local farm since they're in season. If you're looking for fresh blueberries in February, however, they will have to come from the other side of the world. To make it through the long journey, they might require an extra dose of chemicals. Buying locally grown produce that's in season is always best for both your health and the health of the planet.[45]

Watch Out for Emulsifiers

As we engage in global trade, shelf-life issues are met with genius but problematic solutions—namely, pesticides, GMOs, additives, stabilizers, and emulsifiers, among others. This is why the list of ingredients on a bag of shredded cheese doesn't consist of just milk.

You might not have heard of emulsifiers, but I can guarantee you will find them in most of the packaged foods you buy. They're chemicals that enable the homogenization of fats into liquids to keep them from separating. Don't be fooled into thinking that emulsifiers are found only in "junk" food. Many health foods are just as culpable. Emulsifiers are added into lots of foods to improve texture and extend shelf life, including dairy products (yogurt, ice cream, and cheese), nut milks, nut butters, condiments, salad dressings, crackers, and more.

Some of the common bad actors you might find include carrageenan, which induces chronic intestinal inflammation in rodents, while carboxymethylcellulose and polysorbate 80 detrimentally alter intestinal bacteria composition and promote chronic intestinal inflammation.[46]

I spend a lot of time educating my patients about these ingredients. They're often the reason why people continue to suffer from health issues after embracing what they thought was a healthy diet. I wish we could all live in the forest, grow our own food, and avoid these chemicals. Since that isn't possible for most of us, we must do our best to be educated consumers and vote with our wallets.

Avoid Artificial Food Colors

From tomato ketchup to candy to red lipstick, food coloring has been a blessing to food companies because it helps their products look brand new. One of the most commonly used groups of food colorings are called *azo dyes*. They have been used for more than 150 years in textiles and pharmaceuticals as well as food colorings. It's hard to escape them.

Of all the azo dyes, tartrazine is the most allergenic. It can cause symptoms of anxiety, migraines, depression, blurred vision, itching, general weakness, hot sensations, a feeling of suffocation, purple skin patches, and sleep disturbances.[47] Some researchers theorize that it contributes to hyperactivity in children, as well as increased irritability, restlessness, and sleep problems.[48]

In 2010, the Center for Science in the Public Interest published a report called *Food Dyes: A Rainbow of Risks*, which concluded that the nine artificial dyes approved in the United States are likely carcinogenic (which means they cause cancer), and that they cause hypersensitivity reactions and behavioral problems. Food dye consumption has increased fivefold per person since 1955. Three dyes—Red 40, Yellow 5, and Yellow 6—account for 90 percent of the dyes used in foods in the U.S.[49]

I always wondered why food in Europe tastes different, and one reason is that that part of the world has different regulations for food additives. In the United Kingdom, Fanta orange soda is colored with pumpkin and carrot extracts, while the U.S. version uses Red 40 and Yellow 6 dyes. McDonald's strawberry sundaes are colored only with strawberries in Britain, but Red 40 is used in the U.S.[50]

Now that we know safer alternatives do exist and are being used by the same companies in other parts of the world, we need to speak up, spread awareness, and have the dangerous food dyes removed. I'm not saying that orange soda or fast-food strawberry sundaes are healthy, but if you do consume them, you'll be a lot better off without Red 40 and Yellow 6.

Eliminate Artificial Sweeteners

Not too long ago, and even now in many households, people tried to eat a healthier diet by purchasing sugar-free items. Artificial sweeteners such as Equal came on the market in the 1980s and 1990s, but sugar substitutes go back to the late 1800s, when saccharine was discovered. Who could resist the idea of sugary goodies without calories? It seemed like a surefire way to deal with obesity and diabetes. It sounds too good to be true, because it is.

If artificial sweeteners were supposed to be our ticket out of the obesity epidemic, why has the number of people with obesity and diabetes skyrocketed since the 1980s, when artificial sweeteners, GMOs, and fat-free options were introduced? Maybe it's because artificial sweeteners are part of the problem, not the solution.

Despite plenty of studies showing the association between artificial sweeteners and diabetes and obesity,[51] doctors and the American Diabetes Association still promote them as a reasonable weight-loss and sugar-control strategy. No wonder up to 40 percent of Americans still use artificial sweeteners. Yet, the fact that these sweeteners can lead to obesity is not news by any means. Since the 1950s, they have been used in cattle feeds to help animals *gain* weight![52]

Since they contain no calories, it may seem counterintuitive that artificial sweeteners can cause obesity and diabetes, but we've finally figured out the missing part of the equation: the gut microbiome. We now know that artificial sweeteners alter the type of bacteria that grow in the gut. They promote the growth of certain families of bacteria that lead to early signs of diabetes, also known as glucose intolerance.

Researchers took two colonies of mice with the same diet, feeding one group artificial sweeteners and the other with regular sugar. After a few weeks, the mice that were fed artificial sweeteners developed higher blood sugar levels and started gaining weight. Now comes the genius part. The researchers gave the sugar-eating mice an antibiotic, wiped out their gut microbiome, and transplanted them with stool from the mice eating artificial sweeteners. The sugar-eating mice now began developing early signs of diabetes too.[53] Similar findings have been observed in adult humans.

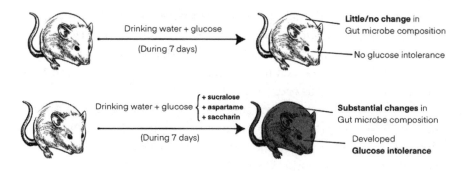

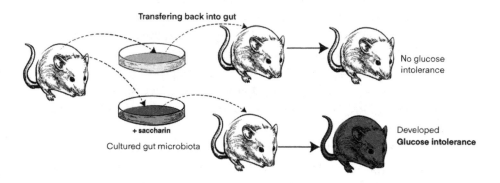

The gut microbiome is a vast universe that we've only recently started exploring. In just the last few decades, it has challenged and changed our understanding of health and diseases. It's about time we start putting the microbiome science into practice to optimize our gut health.

You must be wondering why I haven't said more about probiotic supplementation. It's because the first rule in medicine is "do no harm," and that's far more important and effective than popping a pill. Instead of adding another supplement, it's much more important to make probiotic-rich foods part of our daily diet. Such foods include yogurt, kefir, kombucha, sauerkraut, homemade pickles, miso, tempeh, kimchi, natto made from fermented soybeans, and certain cheeses. Most of my patients love adding yogurt to their diet. However, if you are adding it for the probiotic benefit, make sure the ingredient list says "live active culture." Not all yogurts have living bacteria in them. Also, not all fermented foods have live bacteria. For example, beer is fermented but unfortunately does not count toward your daily dose of probiotics. Many commercially prepared probiotic foods such as pickles and sauerkraut might also be lacking in good bacteria depending on the method used for preparation and preservation.

Prebiotics are also important. These are fiber-rich foods, which are the unsung heroes of the nutrition world. When we eat fiber from a variety of fruits, vegetables, whole grains, and legumes, they feed the good bacteria and keep them happy and proliferating. After all, they are our guests, and a good host always feeds their guests well. Some excellent prebiotic foods include Jerusalem artichoke, onions, leeks, raw banana, dandelion root, asparagus, apple, garlic, and jicama root.

Fecal Microbial Transplantation (FMT)

Many researchers are looking at new drug targets that can change the microbiome itself. One surprising groundbreaking therapy, though, is fecal microbial transplantation. In simple terms, it's a stool transplant from a healthy donor that's injected into a sick patient's colon to add microbial diversity. So far, studies are showing promise in using FMT to treat inflammatory bowel disease (IBD), irritable bowel syndrome (IBS), multiple sclerosis (MS), obesity, insulin resistance, and even certain neuropsychiatric conditions.[54]

Even though FMT might be deemed the latest cutting-edge treatment, it isn't the first time it's been used. Veterinarians were known to use oral or rectal stool therapy to treat animals as long ago as the 17th century.[55] In Ayurveda, enema therapy is the cornerstone of treating almost any condition. In ancient China, fecal content was used to treat acute diarrhea, and patients were fed with "yellow soup."[56] (No surprise, it didn't become popular.)

TIPS FOR PROTECTING YOUR GUT RIGHT NOW

Eating a healthy diet is important for your gut health. However, exposure to hidden culprits can undo all your efforts. That's why I spend a lot of time focusing on gut-protection tips before I even delve into diet itself. Being intentional about what we eat is more than counting calories or worrying about how much protein we are getting. It's far more important to prioritize the "do no harm" strategy when it comes to picking the right foods and leaving the toxic stuff off our plates and out of our pantries. Your gut microbiome will thank you for it.

- Memorize the list of Dirty Dozen produce, and buy the organic ones when possible.

- Wash your produce by soaking it in a solution of baking soda and water or vinegar and water for at least 15 minutes. No more five-second rule!

- Support your community farmers by buying local and seasonal produce when possible.

- Say good-bye to diet foods, along with your stash of artificial sweeteners. Saving a few calories isn't worth compromising your gut microbiome.

- Get in the habit of reading lists of ingredients. If you see carrageenan, carboxymethylcellulose, polysorbate 80, Red 40, Yellow 5, or Yellow 6 in them, put the product back on the shelf and walk away.

- Take antibiotics only when clinically warranted.

- If you must take an antibiotic, add probiotic-rich foods and supplements to your diet while you're taking it—and for at least several weeks afterward.

- Fiber is your best friend because it keeps the good bacteria happy. Nutrition doesn't just consist of carbs, proteins, and fats. Consider fiber your very important fourth food group.

CHAPTER 4

THE DIGESTIVE FIRE

For years, my patient John had been taking acid-blocking medication prescribed by a gastroenterologist. Every time he tried stopping the medication, his symptoms returned. Then over time, in spite of the prescription, his gas, bloating, and loose, frequent stools increased. He didn't know what to do.

His symptoms told me that his digestion was inadequate. When I ran his bloodwork, I found that his vitamin B_{12} and magnesium levels were borderline low. That told me he wasn't absorbing nutrients well.

Was it his diet? Typically, John ate milk and cereal for breakfast, a sandwich with unsweetened iced tea for lunch, popcorn or nuts as a snack, and either chicken or fish with rice and vegetables for dinner. He did have a sweet tooth and would often have ice cream or fruit after dinner, but that wasn't egregious. Plus, to try to keep the heartburn at bay, he had already eliminated coffee, alcohol, and acidic and spicy foods. It seemed like a reasonably healthy American diet, so what was going on? In this chapter, we'll take a careful look at how digestion and metabolism can have a profound impact on overall health.

THE SCIENCE: DIGESTIVE FIRE

You've probably heard the saying "you are what you eat." But that isn't true according to Eastern medicine. What you put in your mouth is a small part of the equation—an important part, but not the only part.

What's even more important is *how* you eat and *how well you digest* your food. Two people can eat the same meal—one with no issues, while the other suffers from gas and bloating. Clearly, what's on their plates isn't necessarily the culprit. The difference between someone who has to unbutton their pants after dinner and someone who doesn't will depend on what I call their "digestive fire," also known as metabolism. This "fire" is responsible for processing the food we eat.

The stronger your fire, the better you can "cook," or digest, the food you eat. In other words, if your fire is strong, you'll have no excessive gas, bloating, or other problems to worry about. On the other hand, if your fire is weak, no matter what you eat—a hamburger or a kale salad—you'll probably have unpleasant digestive symptoms.

Sure, if you're someone who eats fast food every day and drinks soda by the gallon, even a small change in your diet is likely to help you feel a lot better. But few of the patients I see in my practice are in that category. Most are like John—knowledgeable about the basic principles of nutrition and already doing their best to eat a healthy diet. Some of them are even brave (or desperate) enough to stay on highly restricted diets, cutting out gluten and dairy products as well as many fruits, vegetables, and grains. Yet, despite their efforts, they still struggle with symptoms.

As long as what we eat is generally healthy, it makes sense not to emphasize the intake alone. This is why Eastern medicine doesn't subscribe to the concept of a "perfect" diet. What works for one person won't necessarily work for another. According to Ayurveda, properly digested and metabolized food becomes nutrition, while food that isn't metabolized properly becomes toxic. It's all about aligning what you eat with what you can digest.

The bottom line: food is neutral, and how it affects our body depends on our digestive fire. *If our gut isn't functioning optimally, even the best diet won't give us the results we want.*

WHAT GOES WRONG?

With our modern, stressful lifestyles, most of us are victims of weak digestive fire. Instead of a nice stack of dry wood, all we have is some kindling to keep the fire burning.

How do you know if your digestive fire is strong or weak? Note if you have any of these symptoms:

- Lack of hunger or poor appetite
- Sluggishness or sleepiness after eating
- Acid reflux
- Gas and bloating that gets worse as the day progresses
- Dry or sticky stool
- Loose stool with partially digested food
- A white coating on your tongue
- Bad morning breath

While doctors vary in how they diagnose it, this constellation of symptoms is often referred to as irritable bowel syndrome, or IBS. Even if you have only one or two of the above symptoms, your doctor may give you an IBS diagnosis. In that case, your physician may likely send you to a gastroenterologist, who checks you out with a colonoscopy and endoscopy. Then they usually tell you the good news—that you don't have cancer or any other serious condition. "Simply take this acid blocker (or laxative, or fiber), and you'll be fine," they may say. But there's a good chance you still won't be fine after taking these medications.

So you turn to Doctor Google to try to get to the bottom (no pun intended) of the problem. You come across a flurry of diets, supplements, and detox cleanses that promise a flat belly within just a few days. It's hard to resist the sleek marketing, so you open your wallet. Hundreds of dollars later, you might find some relief, but it turns out to be temporary. What now?

If simply eating healthy foods and taking supplements were the key to optimal health, my practice would be rather slow, as anyone following that plan would feel fabulous 24/7. Instead, trying medications, diets, supplements, and cleanses is like buying the very best gas we can find for our old, malfunctioning car without ever fixing its engine. We assume the best quality fuel will make the car run better than before, but you can't make a car fly by filling it with jet fuel. Without the right engine, the fuel has limited value.

I feel for my patients who have struggled so much and endured the most challenging of diets, which sometimes take over their lives, all for nothing but fleeting results. They might feel like they aren't doing enough or are doing something wrong, when the reality is that we're hyperfocused on diet without taking our metabolism into consideration. When we put our focus on the right place—the science—we get the most out of our efforts as we work in sync with our body. This knowledge serves us well, not only for addressing symptoms but also for getting our body back into balance.

First, I concentrate on how the gut works. With that in mind, let's take a look at the first symptom of poor digestion: a poor appetite.

Common Symptom #1: A Poor Appetite

All animals, including humans, are programmed with the basic instinct of hunger. From the minute we're born, we know how to breathe and eat. Eating is critical to our survival as individuals and as a species. If you've ever had an acupuncture treatment, I'll bet you were asked about your appetite. It's an important question in any Eastern medicine assessment because it indicates the strength of our digestive fire.

What happens when we lose our appetite? Does it mean our most fundamental instinct has stopped functioning? Certainly not, yet our fears kick in as if it has. We're so afraid of skipping a meal—even when we have no urge to eat—that we immediately reach for food, certain that not eating will make us weak. Perhaps our body has forgotten about food, we think, so we have to pick up the slack.

It's important to note that there's a difference between appetite and food cravings. Appetite is regulated through a complex interplay between our satiety and hunger hormones called *leptin* and *ghrelin*, respectively. These hormones act as messengers between our gut and brain to tell us when we're hungry and when we've had enough. On the other hand, food cravings are more emotional than physiological. We often get the urge to eat something we like as a reward or a treat. Sometimes, stress makes us crave foods that bring us a sense of comfort. We all have different reasons for food cravings, while our appetite is tightly regulated by our body's needs.

Of course, it can be hard to distinguish true hunger from a craving. One of the ways I help my patients differentiate between the two is to have them notice how they feel after eating. If they feel energized and nourished, they have almost certainly satisfied their hunger and matched their appetite. Their hormones and blood sugar balance out, giving them a feeling of satiety. If they feel sluggish or uneasy after eating, they have probably responded to a craving. This is because the blood sugar and hormones have to work extra hard to balance their metabolism and digest the unexpected food. Over time, my patients learn to tell the difference *before* they eat something.

Many of us in the Western world are fortunate enough to experience real hunger rarely, so it's understandable that we often confuse our cravings for our appetite. If you think about the times when you've lost your appetite while sick, you may recall what it felt like to regain it after a few days of eating very little. *That is true hunger.*

If we come down with the flu, a steak dinner doesn't usually sound so good. This is because the human body is extremely intelligent and efficient. It has a set amount of energy, and it's always figuring out how to conserve it. It carefully prioritizes tasks to allocate our precious resources efficiently. When we're healthy, our digestive fire is strong. We divert energy and blood supply to the gut to help us absorb nutrients and create more energy. In other words, a healthy gut prioritizes digestion and energy generation.

On the other hand, when we're sick, either from an illness or a buildup of too many toxins, our gut's priority shifts. We aren't going to die if we don't eat for a few days, but we might die from an illness or toxins. Therefore, our highly sophisticated body diverts its energy toward fighting infection, reducing inflammation, and eliminating toxins. The principle in this scenario is to conserve energy and prioritize elimination of what might harm the body.

When I ask patients about their appetite, what I'm truly trying to assess is their body's current priority. Option one is to create a strong digestive fire so the patient can absorb nutrients and create more energy. Option two is to focus on fighting any infections, inflammation, or toxins that are getting in the way of a strong digestive fire. How I approach patients in terms of testing, diet, or treatment will differ dramatically based on their answers about appetite. If you find that you're rarely hungry, ask yourself why. Try to understand exactly where your body is spending its energy. This is an important signal that your body gives you.

Common Symptom #2: Sluggishness after Eating

When we get stomach pain, we feel sluggish and unable to focus on anything—possibly for hours. All we want to do is lie down and loosen up our pants a bit. But then, dinnertime rolls around, and we start the cycle all over again. Even when we aren't hungry, we feel obligated to eat three meals a day, because we're used to it. Plus, let's face it, some days, it might be the only fun thing we do.

What happens next? In some cases, instant regret. The digestive system revolts and lets us know that it isn't happy to receive this uninvited workload. The reason we feel so tired after eating is that our body is focusing on digestive tasks, and trying to digest a meal with a weak fire takes a while.

Common Symptom #3: Heartburn and Acid Reflux

You eat a food you love, and suddenly, you struggle to swallow. Pressure comes up from your esophagus and burns, causing pain in your chest that can make it hard to breathe. It's a horrible feeling. We blame stomach acid for this discomfort, but acid actually has a big public relations problem. In truth, we need it to digest our food. Any food we eat has to be broken down into the tiniest pieces so that the nutrients can be absorbed in the gut. If the pieces are too big, the nutrients can't be absorbed. We break down our food somewhat when we chew, but the pieces need to be even smaller for healthy digestion. And we need our stomach acid for that, as well as another secret ingredient called *enzymes*.

You might have heard of one such enzyme called *lactase*. It helps break down the lactose in dairy products. People who are lactose intolerant lack this important enzyme, so when they eat dairy, the lactose remains undigested. It eventually ends up in the colon, where bacteria have a lactose party as they break it down into gas—which often leads to socially challenging flatulence, bloating, and diarrhea. Besides lactase, our pancreas makes a variety of enzymes to help us break down carbohydrates, fats, proteins, and fiber.

The acid in the stomach is an important signal for enzymes to get to work. When we block the acid, we also indirectly block the enzymes. As a result, we can't digest food properly, causing a lot of uncomfortable symptoms from reflux to diarrhea. Not only that, but we also miss out on all those amazing nutrients and vitamins that we need, because we can't absorb them properly.

Stomach acid's vilification has made proton pump inhibitors (PPIs)—medications that block the acid—among the top 10 most prescribed drugs in the world. This isn't surprising, because 25 percent of the population experiences heartburn at least once a month. Unfortunately, while these medications appear to work to alleviate symptoms of acid reflux, or GERD, they cause a lot of damage to the gut microbiome. Studies have found that the use of these medications leads to a significant increase in potentially dangerous pathogenic bacteria. Given the number of people in the world who take them, researchers are concerned that the effects of PPIs on our gut microbiome are more prominent than the effects of antibiotics![1] They're now available over the counter without a warning label about the microbiome, which is a big problem.

Extended use of PPIs (over eight weeks) can cause rebound stomach acid hypersecretions and increased reflux-like symptoms.[2] They can even get in the way of absorption of key vitamins and minerals, leading to higher risk of developing conditions like osteoporosis.[3]

If stomach acid is a good thing, why does it seem to become our enemy at times? Are the cells in the stomach making too much acid? There are very rare conditions that cause certain cells to produce abnormal levels of acid, but none of these are the cause of 99 percent of heartburn cases.

For most of us, our stomach cells do what they're supposed to do, following our cues obediently. The problem is that we give them mixed signals with our diet and certain bad habits. There are three key mistakes we make that studies show have a significant correlation with heartburn and acid reflux:[4]

1. *Irregular mealtimes.* The stomach is a creature of habit. If we eat breakfast around 8 A.M., our stomach starts producing acid and releasing enzymes every day at that time in anticipation of the meal. By the time that avocado toast hits the stomach, it's already showtime, and food is digested easily. Once the job is done, the levels of stomach acid go down until lunch. Now imagine eating at different times every day. The stomach has no heads-up. After our first bite, it has to scramble to get the acid and enzymes into action. The food takes longer to digest, and acid sticks around longer. Of course, we should never eat when we're not actually hungry, whether we have a regular meal schedule or not. So if you aren't hungry at a

regular mealtime, just have water or herbal tea. As you start synchronizing your routine to the circadian rhythm, your hunger is likely to adjust and give you signals at the same times every day.

2. *Snacking and sipping.* If it's hard to find time for a meal, many of us prefer to graze, snack and sip all day. I have patients who adhere to intermittent fasting, so they have nothing but a big cup of black coffee until late afternoon. Others prefer to munch on food rather than have a full meal. But think about it: Do you like to work 24/7? Well, neither does the stomach. The acid-producing cells don't know if the coffee we've sipped or the few nuts we've eaten are supposed to be a meal or a snack. The stomach will release acid and enzymes in response to both, which means it has to work overtime as we graze and sip. It's like begging for heartburn.

3. *Eating too late.* All of that sipping and snacking leaves us hungry at the end of the day, so we try to make up for it with a big, late-night dinner. Just as the stomach was thinking, "Phew! That was a long day of nonstop work," it's called back to the "office" with no promise of overtime pay. Begrudgingly, it gets to work breaking down the food. Then, as we lie down in bed with a belly full of food and no help from gravity, the acid refluxes back into our food pipe. Poor stomach. Not only do we ask it to work overtime, but we ask it to defy the laws of physics.

Ginger tea is great for stimulating digestion, ideally before or with meals. Grate a quarter inch of organic ginger root into boiling water, and let it steep for about five minutes.

Common Symptom #4: Bloated Belly

Bloating isn't just uncomfortable; it also causes the frustrating battle of the bulge. To complicate matters, it can be hard to pinpoint what foods might cause it, as any food can create a different reaction every time we eat it. For instance, nuts are generally good for us. One day, you might have a few almonds with no problem. The next day, a few almonds could cause you to bloat. What are you supposed to do?

Unfortunately, there's no magic pill for bloating or the other common symptoms of IBS. Since it isn't a life-threatening condition, there hasn't been enough research to help us find successful treatments. Yet, I know people who've gone through major depression or had to quit their jobs and end relationships because of IBS symptoms.

An international survey of IBS patients validated its significant impact on their quality of life. To receive a treatment that would make them symptom-free, they said they would give up 25 percent of their remaining life (an average of 15 years), and 14 percent said they'd risk a one-in-a-thousand chance of death.[5] Those are some pretty serious statements, so I pay particular attention to gut complaints.

From the Eastern medicine perspective, bloating, of course, is a sign of weak digestive fire. Bloating is caused by excess gas in the digestive system, but where it's located in that system matters a great deal. When the gas is in the stomach, it can be burped out to provide some relief. When gas is in the large intestine, it might feel better to pass it, either through flatulence or a bowel movement. But before food waste is moved into the large intestine for release, it has to be digested in the small intestine. When the food isn't broken down properly, it remains in the small intestine, and bacteria causes it to ferment. This leads to the production of gas that builds up over time. When gas is trapped in the small intestine, it takes time to come out, so bloating and discomfort result.

Bear in mind that the large intestine is only called "large" because it's bigger in circumference than the "small" one. It's only about five feet long. The so-called "small" intestine, though, is 15 feet long. This means the small intestine has plenty of space for gas to accumulate and show up as bloating.

Additional Symptoms

Besides sluggishness after meals, bloating, and heartburn, there are other less common gastrointestinal complaints I've encountered in my patients. Sometimes they experience sticky stools or loose stools with partially digested food still visible. When they bring these up with their doctors, they often get a shoulder shrug and are asked to eat more fiber.

When the stool is sticky, requiring lots of toilet paper or wipes to clean up, or if you see partially digested food, it once again points to a weak digestion. Sticky stools can be due to poor fat digestion and absorption, whereas partially digested food could be a consequence of not chewing properly combined with low acid and enzyme levels in the stomach.

Other symptoms I've noticed are bad morning breath, along with a thick, white coating on the tongue. The microbiome of your mouth is very much connected with the bacteria in your gut, as we discussed before. In Eastern medicine, the tongue reflects your gut—especially your colon. Bad morning breath and a coating on the tongue can indicate buildup of old stool in the gut, often seen with chronic constipation. It can also point to an imbalance between good and bad bacteria, along with possible yeast overgrowth.

Solutions to all these common symptoms aren't simple, as you have to try different strategies to find what works for you. I've found that my patients respond well to the suggestions in the next section, because these techniques strengthen our digestive fire.

THE SOLUTION: STRENGTHEN YOUR DIGESTION

You may have heard these suggestions before, but most people I meet don't realize how important these solutions are for strengthening their digestion. While your conventional doctor or even your mother may have recommended one or more of these to you, they're basic principles of Eastern medicine. Let's explore just why they're so important for your digestive fire.

Avoid Overeating

While you might have been instructed as a child to eat everything on your plate, overeating isn't good for anyone. But it can be particularly detrimental to people with weak digestion. Since they don't have enough acid or enzymes in the stomach to break down that much food, eating too much overwhelms their digestive capacity.

Every day in my practice, I treat the consequences of overconsumption. Yet, surprisingly, I see more nutritional deficiencies in people who consume more calories than their body needs. This is because calories don't necessarily equal nutrition. According to Ayurveda, anything in excess of what your body needs is poison—especially food. When we eat in moderation, the food is digested well and turns into nutrition, while anything that isn't digested becomes a toxin.

To get an idea of your stomach's capacity, cup your palms together. Your stomach is about the size of a ball that would fit in your palms. If you look at the portions you're served at the average restaurant, it's easy to see why there's a problem.

Your stomach's gastric juices are made up of its acid and enzymes. The total amount of gastric juices needed to digest a full meal can be as much as 32 ounces! When I explain this concept to my patients, I often use the washing machine analogy. Let's say you're about to do a load of laundry to wash your dirty gym clothes. You need water—probably hot water—to get the grime out, along with detergent. But what if you overstuff the washer with clothes? There's not enough room for the water and detergent, and the clothes won't get shaken well enough to come clean. That's the reason we fill the washer only two-thirds to three-quarters of its capacity. The same concept applies to our stomachs. We should eat only until we're about two-thirds to three-quarters full, leaving enough room for the digestive juices to work their magic. When we overeat, food is forced out of the stomach prematurely. If you experience burping, overeating especially will be your enemy. To make room in the overstuffed stomach, the air gets pushed up and out as a belch. Sometimes, when we eat a lot of food too quickly, we get cramps, which are stomach spasms that occur as it tries to empty in a hurry.

When food doesn't get digested, it's like an unlimited buffet for the bacteria who will happily chow down on the leftovers, leaving us gassy and bloated. In my experience, more than half of bloating issues can be remedied by simply eating half the portion of food we normally eat. This isn't about cutting calories; it's about not stuffing the stomach too full.

If you're skeptical, just try it. Consume only 50 percent of the food you normally eat at any given meal. I'll bet you'll be shocked to find that you actually feel more energetic afterward, not lethargic. Also, you probably won't have the usual gas and bloating issue, and you'll feel lighter on your toes. That's what happens when you work *with* your body's functioning rather than against it. And if you've learned to distinguish between hunger and appetite, as we discussed earlier, you'll also learn when your stomach is telling you it's full.

Remember that small, easy-to-digest meals will keep your digestive fire going strong for the next meal without putting you in a food coma. No matter what, match your food intake to how hungry you truly feel. That way you won't overwhelm your already weak digestion with more than you can process.

Don't Drink Water with Meals, Especially Cold Water

Let's say you go out for dinner at a restaurant in America. It's common for the waitstaff to come over, greet you, and take your drink order. While you wait for your drink, you're usually served a big glass of ice water. Since you're hungry and probably thirsty—because many of us forget to hydrate enough during the day—you start drinking this water as you wait for your meal. If overeating is like stacking too much wood on a fire and suffocating it, drinking too much water with your meal is like putting the fire out unintentionally.

The stomach acid and enzymes become diluted significantly by this onslaught of water in an empty stomach. Not only that, but the water takes up precious real estate inside. Some people even believe that if you fill your stomach with water first, you'll end up eating less. But this is not a smart weight-loss strategy. Drinking a bit of water with meals is fine and can help with digestion, but ideally, most of your water intake should happen *between* meals.

That's the water part of the problem. But ice is also a culprit. Particularly in the U.S., we think of water as water, regardless of its temperature. However, if you've traveled to Europe or Asia, you've probably noticed an absence of ice. One of the things that surprised me when I was at the Singapore airport was that there were hot water stations all over the place. Given that the average temperature there is a steamy 90 degrees, this abundance of hot water and lack of ice machines seemed odd. Contrast that to the airport in Miami where you have ice-cold water and other beverages available every few steps.

You don't even have to travel to Asia to see this trend. Go to any authentic Asian restaurant, and one of the first things served to you will be tea in tiny cups. The purpose of this small amount of hot tea at the beginning of the meal is to stimulate digestion. This is also why soup is often the first course of a meal. It's warm and easy to process, ramping up digestion to get the stomach ready for the entrée.

Anytime you put something warm in the stomach, it increases blood circulation, which helps ramp up the production of digestive juices. In contrast, anything cold in the stomach constricts the blood vessels and slows digestion. When you go out in a blizzard, your hands and face turn pale, but on a hot summer day, your face becomes flushed. Blood rushes toward heat and away from cold.

Eating warm foods is often more satisfying, and they are easier to digest. When I have patients who struggle with gastrointestinal symptoms such as constipation, diarrhea, gas, or bloating, I often instruct them to opt for warm, liquid foods like soups and stews rather than cold, dry foods like sandwiches. Warm, liquid foods help to move all food through your system.[6] They're gentler on your stomach and ensure better absorption of nutrients.

Other regions in the world also have a tradition of drinking something at the beginning of the meal to aid digestion. In Europe, you're likely to be served an aperitif before your meal. Aperitifs such as liqueur, vermouth, spirits, and bitters are often low in alcohol content. They are flavored with local herbs, fruits, flowers, and spices. Even wine can help with digestion. For anyone who has traveled to Europe, you might have realized that a bottle of water is sometimes more expensive than a glass of wine. Henceforth, you can follow doctor's orders and enjoy an aperitif or a glass of wine with your meal rather than a large glass of ice water.

Chew Food Properly

A common piece of advice is to chew food 32 times,[7] not just two or three. The act of chewing mechanically breaks down food into smaller pieces so that it's easier to digest. All too often, we eat mindlessly, chewing just enough to avoid choking. As poorly broken-down food passes through, the stomach has its work cut out for it. Since the stomach doesn't have teeth, it has to use chemicals. When it's bombarded with large chunks of food, it must work overtime again, and it needs more acid and enzymes to get the job done.

Even with extra acid, some of the food won't get digested, which leads to more of the unsavory symptoms we've been talking about—like acid reflux, gas, bloating, constipation, or diarrhea.

Chewing lends the stomach a hand, while it also helps us feel more satiated, reducing hunger and helping us absorb more nutrients.[8]

When we take our time with chewing our food, it allows our brain enough of a chance to get the right signals from the stomach about feeling full. We end up eating less and feeling more satiated. Properly digested food is also easier for the gut to extract nutrients from. After all, if we're trying to eat healthy, we want to glean every ounce of nutrition from it. There's no point in pooping out all our effort and money.

> Cumin, coriander, and fennel tea (CCF tea) is good to drink with or after a meal. It helps stimulate digestion while minimizing gas and bloating symptoms. Add one teaspoon of each to boiling water and let the mixture steep for five minutes. Enjoy!

THE FODMAP DIET

While I've said it isn't about *what* you eat and that Eastern medicine doesn't subscribe to any particular diet, there are certain dietary changes that help most people avoid gas and bloating. I ask patients with those symptoms to try the low-FODMAP diet. *FODMAP* stands for "fermentable oligosaccharides, disaccharides, monosaccharides, and polyols."

Studies have shown that the low-FODMAP diet helps 50 to 80 percent of patients with IBS, especially in relieving bloating, flatulence, and diarrhea. It also leads to profound positive changes in the gut microbiome.[9] The concept here is the same as Eastern medicine's: foods that are easier to digest will cause less gas and bloating. The low-FODMAP diet reduces the types of foods that contain easily fermentable sugars, which typically lead to more gastrointestinal symptoms in someone with weak digestion.

Many of the foods listed as high FODMAP are considered healthy. However, they confer their health benefits only if they are digested properly. For instance, cauliflower is very good for us.

However, if you are someone who experiences a lot of gas after eating cauliflower, it's best for you to avoid it. There are plenty of other foods on the low-FODMAP list that still offer the nutrients you need. Here's a handy list of high- and low-FODMAP foods from Monash University in Australia.[10]

	High FODMAP Foods to avoid	Low FODMAP Eat this instead
Vegetables	Artichokes, asparagus, cauliflower, garlic, green peas, mushrooms, onions, sugar snap peas	Eggplant, green beans, bok choy, bell pepper, carrots, cucumbers, lettuce, potatoes, zucchini
Fruits	Apples, cherries, dried fruit, mango, nectarines, peaches, pears, plums, watermelon	Cantaloupe, kiwi fruit (green), mandarin, orange, pineapple
Dairy & alternatives	Cow's milk, ice cream, soy milk, condensed milk, yogurt	Almond milk, brie/camembert cheese, feta cheese, hard cheeses, lactose-free milk
Protein sources	Most legumes/pulses, some marinated meats/poultry/seafood (marinade might contain garlic, onions), processed meats	Eggs, tofu, plain cooked meats/poultry/seafood, tempeh
Breads & cereals	Wheat/rye/barley-based breads, breakfast cereals, cookies, and snack products	Corn flakes, oats, quinoa flakes, quinoa/rice/corn pasta, rice cakes (plain), sourdough spelt bread, wheat/rye/barley-free breads
Sugars, sweeteners	High-fructose corn syrup, honey, sugar-free desserts	Dark chocolate, maple syrup, rice malt syrup, table sugar
Nuts & seeds	Cashews, pistachios	Macadamias, peanuts, pumpkin seeds/pepitas, walnuts

I realize that the low-FODMAP diet can be challenging. It isn't the easiest or most intuitive plan. Fortunately, with rising awareness, there are many apps and cookbooks that can make it simpler to follow. I even recommend a food delivery service to my patients that makes gluten-free, low-FODMAP meals. This comes in handy when you don't have time to cook.

Key Ayurvedic Tips for Digestion

General Nutritional Therapy of Ayurveda	Dos	Don'ts
Warm	Eat 2 to 3 warm meals per day Enjoy fresh fruits once a day	Bread Raw vegetables Food or beverages directly from the fridge
Regular	*Breakfast:* Keep it light, avoid skipping *Lunch:* The main meal of the day *Dinner:* Early—between 6 and 7 P.M.	Irregular meals Snacking Eating late at night
Light in digestion but well nourishing	Plant-based proteins (nuts, seeds, beans, lentils, tofu, tempeh, seitan, whole-grain cereals) Plant-based fats (olive oil, sesame oil, ghee/clarified butter, coconut oil)	Animal protein (meat, poultry, fish) Fatty or deep-fried foods Ice cream Desserts Cheese Yogurt (especially in the evening)
High-quality and fresh foods	Preferably organic and/or locally grown Freshly prepared as often as possible	Highly processed food Fast food Frozen meals Commercial soft drinks

In addition to the low-FODMAP diet, I also incorporate several personalized recommendations based in Ayurvedic medicine. This approach matches foods to the strength of each individual's digestive fire. For instance, someone with a lot of IBS symptoms and weak digestion should probably avoid rare steak for dinner, opting instead for a vegetable stew with quinoa.

The Ayurvedic approach also incorporates other important lifestyle changes that teach us not only what to eat but also how to eat. In my opinion, combining the low-FODMAP diet with Ayurvedic intervention is often a win-win.

It didn't surprise me when a recent randomized controlled trial in Germany demonstrated what I've seen in my practice. This study compared the low-FODMAP diet to the Ayurvedic approach. What it found was that in just three months, IBS symptom reduction was significantly higher and more clinically meaningful in the Ayurvedic group compared to the group that followed the low-FODMAP diet alone.[11]

KEEPING YOUR DIGESTION STRONG

In Eastern medicine, diet is customized for each individual based on what their body is able to process. Eating what we can digest is the key to gut health. You already know there are days when you aren't particularly hungry and feel bloated or constipated. Those are the days when you should eat light, easy-to-digest foods rather than a steak dinner. Imagine trying to turn a steak into mush (aka poop). It requires a lot of work. On the other hand, a stew with vegetables and quinoa or rice is much easier for the stomach to handle.

The temperature, consistency, and quantity of food can be our ally in keeping our gut happy, as well as the qualities of our food—not just how many carbs or proteins we eat.

When I discuss these topics with my patients like John, the man you read about at the beginning of the chapter, the information is often contradictory to everything they've been told before. Yet, these Ayurvedic principles apply the facts of chemistry and physics to our own bodies and make sense to my patients.

For John, we changed his diet to support his digestion, which was affected by the acid-blocking medication he'd been taking. Our goal was to have him come off the medication, but we had to do it slowly to prevent rebound symptoms. His new diet plan included warm steel-cut oatmeal in the morning with stewed fruits. For lunch, he had soup and salad, along with a cup of fennel tea. As a snack, he ate some fruit, but only if he was hungry. Dinner was the same as usual for him, but a smaller portion. His last meal of the day was always four hours before bedtime, and he stopped eating ice cream after dinner. Instead, he had a cup of marshmallow-root or chamomile tea. We added certain supplements such as digestive enzymes to help break down his food and prevent gas, bloating, and diarrhea. We also used certain herbs and teas that helped balance the acid and soothe the stomach lining.

After nine months, John was able to stop taking the acid-blocking medication that had been a part of his life for more than seven years. As his digestive fire was optimized, he stuck to the regimen because he felt so much better. He also noted that he had more energy and slept more soundly. During the day, he was no longer sluggish after meals and was able to stay sharp and focused at work without relying on caffeine to make it through.

TIPS FOR RELIEVING YOUR SYMPTOMS AND STRENGTHENING YOUR DIGESTIVE FIRE

Here are some tips to help you feel more aligned with your body by keeping your digestive fire strong:

1. Eat two to three meals per day, separated by at least three to four hours. The heavier the meal, the longer it takes to digest.

2. Chew your food well—at least 30 times before swallowing.

3. Eat food portions that take up only 75 percent of your capacity. The price we pay for the extra 25 percent in the form of gas, bloating, and heartburn isn't worth it.

4. While eating, get in the habit of either expressing gratitude for the meal or taking a moment to appreciate the look and smell of the food.

5. Avoid cold foods and beverages, since they slow digestion.

6. Avoid gluten, dairy products, and raw vegetables if you have weak digestion, or at least until your digestive fire improves.

7. Limit your liquid intake to one cup of room-temperature water with your meals. You can also opt for an herbal tea with or after your meal to stimulate your digestion.

8. Most of your water intake should be between meals, ideally an hour before or after a meal. Mealtimes are meant for eating food, not drinking water.

9. Avoid snacking between meals to allow your stomach to replenish its stores of acid and enzymes. Even your stomach has rights! Don't expect it to work more than eight hours a day without a break.

10. Since nighttime is for sleeping, not digesting a meal, dinner should be finished at least four hours prior to bedtime.

11. Last, but not least, *eat only when hungry.*

CHAPTER 5

THE ROOT CAUSE

Have you ever been so inspired by a diet success story that you decided to try the same diet? Maybe you and your loved one followed it together. Somehow, your partner lost weight, but your scale barely moved. Most of us have been there. With a never-ending buffet of diets in fashion one day and out of fashion the next, many people have been through a revolving door of diet plans. There's a reason, though, why a plan might work for the person with the success story but not for you.

Each of us is a product of our genetics, environment, microbiome, diet, and lifestyle. One person might even be given the same diagnosis as another, but their health journey is unique to them. We are so much more than our diagnoses.

My patient Sam is a case in point. When I met him, his symptoms were making him miserable. He described feeling like he was "overheating inside and out." He suffered from an autoimmune condition called *scleroderma*, which affected his gut, skin, joints, and even his lungs. For months, he had suffered with his most recent symptoms—burning in his stomach and diarrhea. He'd tried everything from medications to drastic dietary changes, but nothing helped.

To truly understand what was happening with Sam, I had to use my private investigation talents to determine the *root cause* of his symptoms. I loved reading mystery novels when I was growing up, and I dreamed of becoming Hercule Poirot or Sherlock Holmes. While I'll never become a PI, my profession puts me in a position to search for clues, gather evidence, and come up with the most plausible explanation of how the series of events that led to the "crime" unfolded. I also try to figure out the motive.

Of course, in medicine the "crime" is the disease or symptom, while the "crime scene" is the body itself. The "motive" (or the "why") is the root cause of the symptoms or disease. I must seek out clues through blood tests, scans, and a thorough assessment of each patient. It's painstaking detective work that takes time, but it's well worth it to bring my patients relief.

What I learned in medical school, however, was more straightforward than this. I was to match a group of symptoms to a diagnosis and prescribe a specific set of medications that were meant to treat it. I wasn't trained to connect the dots and re-create a sequence of events for my patients. Who could be bothered with explaining complex pathophysiology to someone with no medical knowledge? It worked out in most cases, since people expected to receive a diagnosis—and a pill to go with it.

This is why, from a Western medicine perspective, it was difficult for Sam's doctors to treat his symptoms. Every medication they prescribed caused side effects that led to more prescriptions. It was turning into a game of *Whac-A-Mole*. For many patients, like Sam, this "one size fits all" approach simply doesn't work. We have to dig deeper and pull out our proverbial magnifying glass.

THE SCIENCE: THE ROOT CAUSE

The first step to determining the root cause of a symptom or disease is to learn whether our digestive fire is strong or weak—and therefore, if our metabolism is strong or weak. Until we know this, it's like turning on the oven to cook dinner but having no idea what temperature it is set at. My patients often make the mistake of trying to figure out what to eat before they learn what they can properly digest and metabolize. No wonder so many people try lots of diets before they find one that works (if they ever find one).

It makes more sense to put the horse before the cart—learning the strength or weakness of your digestive fire and metabolism so that you can pick a diet to match. If your oven can go up to only 300 degrees, maybe roasting a whole turkey is not a good idea. Once you know what your metabolism is like, you can learn how to choose the right food to help it run optimally. When I know the types of imbalances to which a particular patient's body is prone, I can help them define the diet that will work best for them.

Those of us with a strong digestive fire and metabolism can usually get away with eating anything if it falls in the healthy category. Those of us with a weaker digestive fire and metabolism must be more intentional about what we choose to eat.

Even Western medicine is finally coming to terms with the fact that we're all unique, with different metabolisms. This explains the new field of precision medicine, which seeks to develop diagnostics and therapeutics that consider individual variability in environment, lifestyle, genetics, and our molecular makeup.[1] Our metabolism is a product of thousands of chemical reactions that take place within a cell. As a result of these reactions, numerous small molecules are produced in the body. Think of them as our unique metabolic fingerprint. Just like our genes make up our genome, these tiny molecules make up our "metabolome."

But while our genes don't change, our metabolism does. Therefore, looking at your unique metabolome can give you real-time insight into how your body is functioning. There are many factors that directly impact this process. Researchers are investigating the interplay between our genes, diet, lifestyle, environment, microbiome, and their effects on our metabolism.[2] I hope it now makes perfect sense why I've been discussing the circadian rhythm, good bacteria, the digestive fire, and now diet. All these unique components make up who we are.

These inherent differences between us are why there's no such thing as a "perfect" diet, according to Eastern medicine. Instead, the practitioner strives to figure out the strength of the patient's digestive fire and metabolome in order to prescribe foods that will match. If someone presents with specific symptoms or a disease, the practitioner will also investigate the root cause. This helps them decipher the patient's tendencies toward certain imbalances. All this information is then assembled into a customized treatment plan. That certainly sounds like precision medicine to me.

Since most of us have a weak digestive fire and metabolism, we need help to choose the right diet. But again, it's more complicated than simply eating foods that have been deemed "healthy."

WHAT GOES WRONG?

As much as people in my profession would like to believe that we have an answer for everything, we just don't. Very often, we're stumped by the most common symptoms and don't have answers to even simple questions. I wish every patient I saw was like one on an episode of the TV show *House* about the doctor who diagnosed difficult cases. They would show up with a mysterious, yet classic symptom that would neatly fit into a box labeled "rare disease." Unfortunately, real life is a bit more complex and nuanced than that.

The truth is that most doctors cringe when they encounter symptoms like fatigue, insomnia, body aches, irritable bowel syndrome, hair loss, and anxiety. There are pills for these symptoms, but most patients have tried them all, with little to no improvement. These somewhat vague but prevalent symptoms are much harder to address than someone who shows up with, say, green urine.

On the other side of the exam table is the patient who has been living with these symptoms for far too long. All they're asking for are answers and relief. They place their hopes in one specialist after another and one pill after another. Once their doctors run out of medications to prescribe, the patient is pretty much out of luck—and has potentially done more damage to their body.

The next step is likely a referral to a psychiatrist. Since no lab or radiology test can figure out what's wrong, the profession assumes it must be in the patient's head. "You're probably just depressed," they might say. If only I had a penny for every time a patient told me they'd heard this from a doctor! If no doctor can figure out what's wrong with you or how to help you feel better, wouldn't you be depressed?

I appreciate my extensive medical training, but I prefer the Sherlock Holmes route. Most of the time, I won't end up with a clear-cut diagnosis, but I can certainly piece together why and how the disease came about. This can help me as a medical provider to pick the best treatment and diet, helping the patient obtain some relief and closure. It also gives them confidence in our therapeutic relationship. This is why I firmly believe that the Eastern medicine approach to identifying the root cause of any disease is still as relevant today as it was thousands of years ago.

An Imbalance of Yin and Yang

In traditional Chinese medicine (TCM), the belief is that a state of health signifies the balance of yin and yang, while a disease state implies an imbalance.[3] These two energetically opposite forces work synergistically to create equilibrium. When we get sick, it's usually because there's too much or too little yin or yang. The balance we're trying to attain and maintain is with ourselves and our environment. If we're in harmony with nature, it's easier to bring our body back into balance.

To figure out what has caused the imbalance, TCM identifies the root cause as either external or internal. External causes are related to the environment and are often out of our control, such as the weather or pathogens. Internal causes stem from our choices with regard to diet, sleep, stress level, and activity level. All these in turn have a positive or negative influence on our mind and body. Luckily, internal causes are often under our control. We can decide how to nourish our body, how much we exercise, how much sleep we get, and how we manage our stress levels. Intentional health is all about bringing awareness to these internal and external influences, and knowing the root cause of our problems makes it much easier to find a solution.

External Causes of Imbalance

An imbalance due to an external, environmental factor disrupts the delicate milieu of the five elements: earth, water, fire, air, and ether. This could be anything from an infection to an extreme weather event, which can lead to too much heat or cold, or rain or drought.

Thousands of years ago, severe weather and untreatable infections posed threats to our ancestors' health. Today, man-made threats are among the main causes of health imbalances. Since we live in an era of climate change, all these phenomena will continue to have a significant impact on our health. Unfortunately, our health-care system is ill prepared to deal with these threats. According to the CDC, the health effects of these disruptions in our physical, biological, and ecological systems include increased respiratory and cardiovascular disease, injuries, premature deaths related to extreme weather events, changes in the prevalence and geographical distribution of food- and water-borne illnesses and other infectious diseases, and threats to mental health.[4]

Air pollution alone is now the biggest environmental risk for early death, according to the Environmental Defense Fund. It's responsible for more than six million premature deaths each year from heart attacks, strokes, diabetes, and respiratory diseases. That's more than the deaths from AIDS, tuberculosis, and malaria combined.[5]

Any time I make diet recommendations, I always try to consider the external environmental impact of our food choices. The blood and urine tests I use analyze heavy metals and other pollutants as part of the assessment. Living and practicing medicine in a big city like New York particularly requires a customized environmental risk assessment. According to a study, New Yorkers have been found to have mercury levels more than three times the national levels—almost a quarter of the NYC adult population had blood mercury concentration at or above the five-micrograms-per-liter New York State reportable level.[6]

If you live in New York City, there's a one-in-four chance that your heavy metal levels are higher than they should be. Today, as people try to avoid eating meat, they often turn to seafood as a healthier alternative, which can increase their exposure to heavy metals like mercury. We should monitor this closely—but I'll bet your doctor has never checked your heavy metal levels. This is just one of the ways in which Western medicine isn't prepared to deal with the environmental impact on our health.

Every time I see patients with a history of cancer, especially breast cancer, I educate them about how the environment affects their health. In the absence of significant family history, environmental factors can be the root cause. For instance, studies have suggested a link between increased risk of breast cancer and exposure to bisphenols such as BPA, even at doses below what the U.S. Food and Drug Administration (FDA) considers safe for consumption.[7]

Unfortunately, BPA is everywhere. Plastic water bottles, food packaging, canned foods, IV tubing, and even store receipts are coated with this chemical. Its composition is similar to estrogen, and it binds the estrogen receptors in our body, causing the cells to proliferate: a recipe for cancer.[8] There are ways to measure BPA in our urine to get an idea of the level of exposure. In my practice, a simple environmental questionnaire can give me a good idea of the level of someone's exposure based on the foods they eat, as well as the types of cleaning and personal hygiene products they use.

Even small, intentional changes in our exposure can make a big difference. Switching to a diet that avoids foods that come in cans or plastic packaging can reduce urinary levels of BPA by 65 percent in just three days,[9] and this impact can add up. Besides breast cancer, many other hormonal conditions such as thyroid disease and polycystic ovary syndrome (PCOS) also warrant a closer look at the chemicals lurking in the products we use daily.

Examining these environmental factors has helped me uncover hidden causes of several ailments that patients have suffered from for years.

Internal Causes of Imbalance

Whenever I see a patient, besides evaluating their digestive fire and metabolism, I look at the four key domains of their health: diet, sleep, exercise, and stress management. Any disruptions in these will lead to diseases in the future, so they're the main internal causes of imbalance. Once I know which domain is out of balance, I can shift my focus toward it and dig deeper. In this chapter, we will take a closer look at the role our diet plays in striking a good balance.

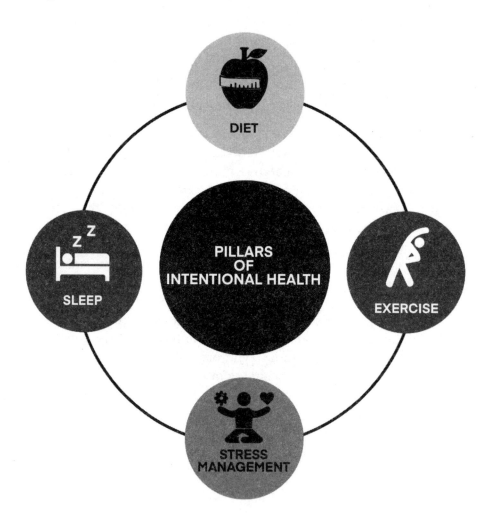

An Imbalance in Your Constitution

Diet is one of the four important domains or pillars of intentional health. To help customize a diet for a patient, I determine one of their key physical qualities: their "constitution." Think of this as the set of genetic tendencies with which they were born that influence the type of imbalance they're most likely to develop. For instance, some people get sinus infections and allergies easily, always battling a runny nose and watering eyes. Others have dry eyes and a dry nose. Similarly, some people are prone to constipation and gas, while others are more likely to have acid reflux and diarrhea.

What determines these tendencies? Western medicine calls it "genetic predisposition," while Eastern medicine attributes it to different constitutions. This explains why eating a certain diet works for some people but not others. Getting to know your constitution can be helpful in preventing diseases and alleviating symptoms.

Eastern medicine has simplified the concept of determining your constitution by evaluating four basic categories: hot, cold, damp, and dry. Most of us are a combination of hot or cold along with either damp or dry. It might seem silly at first to associate our genetic tendencies with these terms, but I believe you'll understand it once I explain further.

A couple thousand years ago, Hippocrates concurred with these concepts. "In men, all diseases are caused by bile and phlegm when they become too dry or too wet or too hot or too cold in the body." He further said such changes were brought about by food, drink, exercise, wounds, senses, sex, and the weather.[10]

In Chinese medicine, the same concept exists. Its diet and lifestyle recommendations are based on our constitution. This concept also explains why we might do better in one season than another. Some people who run hot suffer from more heartburn in the summer versus the winter. Someone who has a dry constitution might have worsening constipation during the cold and dry winter months. The overall weather pattern of where we live also has a significant influence on our health. For instance, someone who has a hot and dry constitution might not do well in a desert like Arizona but will thrive in cool and damp Seattle. On the

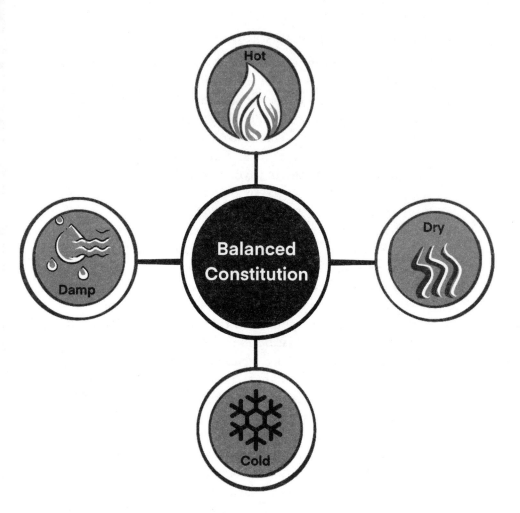

other hand, someone who is always congested might do better in Arizona than Seattle.

Similarly, our constitution might be affected based on the season or the type of climate we live in. Everyone has a favorite season when they feel their best and another time in the year when they feel not so great. I personally love spring and am not a fan of cold weather. Because of my "cold" constitution, I prefer a warmer climate and warmer foods. When winter comes around, I pay particular attention to getting an extra dose of self-care. Whether it's drinking warm teas or spending time in the sauna, knowing my constitution helps me be proactive about my health.

It's much easier to get to the root cause of any ailment when we have a better understanding of our constitution. Then we can deduce how external and internal causes of imbalance will naturally affect it. In addition to digestive fire and metabolism, I use this information to figure out which diet and lifestyle changes are most appropriate for my individual patients, along with a seasonal adaptation of their food choices to help their body stay in balance.

Let's explore what happens when our body has too much heat, cold, dampness, or dryness.

Common Symptom #1: Too Much Heat

Earlier in the chapter, I mentioned Sam, who described feeling hot "inside and out." He felt like his whole body was inflamed. In traditional Chinese medicine, too much heat in the body can manifest as inflammation. This can lead to more than one "itis," such as dermatitis (inflammation of the skin), arthritis (inflammation of the joints), or colitis or gastritis (inflammation of the gut). Sam was experiencing almost all of these. He was indeed "on fire." Fire does not always mean you feel hot all the time. You can feel cold and still have symptoms of too much "heat" or inflammation.

People with this kind of excess heat often suffer from acid reflux, acne, skin rashes, excessive sweating, anger, irritability, and a bitter or sour taste in their mouth. Heat is often associated with excess yang energy or not enough yin energy in the body.

Conditions associated with excess heat include:

- Skin: dermatitis, rashes, acne
- Joints and muscles: arthritis, painful swollen joints
- Gut: acid reflux, ulcers, gastritis, colitis
- Other: high blood pressure, headaches, cystitis, sinusitis, excessive sweating
- Emotions: anger, irritability, frustration

Common Symptom #2: Too Much Cold

The opposite of too much heat is too much cold, which is characterized by not enough yang or too much yin energy. It often manifests as poor circulation, cold extremities, feeling cold all the time, and slow digestion.

Conditions associated with excess "cold" include:

- Skin: paleness, dryness
- Joints and muscles: stiffness, pain
- Gut: constipation, bloating, slow digestion
- Other: cold extremities, poor circulation
- Emotions: lack of energy and motivation

Common Symptom #3: Too Much Dampness

The concept of feeling dampness in the body might seem a bit abstract. The best way to describe it is the sensation caused by an overload of fluid or mucus. People who tend to develop dampness often suffer from swollen legs, a puffy face, a stuffy nose, chronic congestion, and/or allergies. They feel heaviness and stagnation. People who live in a cold, wet climate are often susceptible to developing dampness symptoms. Since those with this constitution have a slow metabolism, they can also gain weight easily.

Conditions associated with excess "dampness" include:

- Skin: puffiness, swelling
- Joints and muscles: stiffness, pain, swelling
- Gut: constipation with sticky stool, bloating, slow digestion
- Other: tendency to retain fluid, easy weight gain, mucus, congestion
- Emotions: depression, sluggishness

Common Symptom #4: Too Much Dryness

This one is easy to understand. People with a tendency to experience dryness have dry skin, concentrated urine (urine containing a high concentration of dissolved particles), a dry cough, and brittle nails and hair, and they feel dehydrated and depleted easily. They also tend to suffer from constipation with dry, hard stools. Living in a hot, dry climate can exacerbate these symptoms. If their diet consists of "drying" foods, they might experience a lot of gas and bloating.

Conditions associated with excess "dryness" include:

- Skin: dryness, thinning, wrinkles
- Joints and muscles: cracking joints, osteoarthritis
- Gut: gas, constipation with dry, hard stool; bloating
- Other: dry cough; dark, concentrated urine; hair loss; dry nails
- Emotions: anxiety, fear

THE SOLUTION: EAT FOR YOUR CONSTITUTION

Here's a simple quiz to help you determine your constitution. Check each bullet point that applies, and add up your score in each section to find whether you tend to be hot versus cold or damp versus dry. There can be some overlap, however, that may make your outcome less than definitive. In that case, focus on the symptoms that are more pronounced and chronic. This chart is simply a tool to narrow down your constitution. As you continue reading, you'll learn how to apply your score to your diet.

HOT	COLD	DAMP	DRY
❏ I feel hot very easily	❏ I feel cold very easily	❏ I sweat easily	❏ I feel dry often
❏ I prefer a cooler climate	❏ I prefer a warmer climate	❏ I prefer a dry climate	❏ I prefer a humid climate
❏ I have a strong appetite	❏ I have a weak appetite	❏ I sometimes get swelling in my legs	❏ I have dry eyes and mouth
❏ I like to be active	❏ I get tired easily	❏ I feel congested often with a runny nose	❏ I get dehydrated easily
❏ I have an outgoing personality	❏ I have a reserved personality	❏ My skin and hair can get oily	❏ My hair can be dry and brittle
❏ My face gets flushed often	❏ My hands and feet are usually cold	❏ I gain weight easily	❏ I feel anxious often and tend to worry more
❏ My tongue is usually red	❏ My tongue is pale	❏ My tongue has a white coating	❏ I tend to get constipated easily
❏ I tend to get angry or frustrated easily	❏ I tend to feel down often	❏ I sometimes lack motivation to do things	❏ My tongue is often dry and cracked
Total Score	Total Score	Total Score	Total Score

Understand Food Energetics

In Western medicine, we often think of diet in terms of carbs, proteins, fats, and vitamins. We like to dissect the chemical makeup of foods to determine if they're "healthy" or not. Eastern medicine has a more holistic and even poetic view of what constitutes "healthy" food. That's because the food we eat is far more than just its chemical makeup. The type of environment where it grew determines how it affects our body after we eat it.

Looking beyond chemical composition, Eastern medicine focuses on the energetic properties of foods. For example, Chinese medicine believes the air we breathe, the water we drink, and the food we eat are transformed into qi, or energy, that nourishes us. The energetics of each food have a direct impact on how it's metabolized in our body. As much as I account for the right balance of carbohydrates, proteins, fats, and vitamins in someone's diet, I also teach my patients the concept of food energetics. This is why supposedly healthy diets don't work for some people.

Just as with our constitution, the energetic properties of hot, cold, damp, and dry can also be applied to foods. In other words, some have more yang energy, and others have more yin. One is not better than the other. *Instead, remember that striking a balance between these energetic forces is the key to intentional health.*

Most of us aren't used to thinking about our food as heat-producing or cooling, but bear in mind that I'm not talking about the literal temperature of the food as I did in the last chapter. While literal temperature is important, in this case, it's about the energy. For example, certain foods can have a warming effect, so if we overdo them, they can lead to inflammation. It's an even stranger concept to most of us that certain foods can cause dampness or mucus buildup, while others can lead to dryness.

As poetic as this concept may be, there's science to back it up. A systematic review of 13 randomized controlled trials (RCTs) with more than 4,695 patients evaluated whether the traditional Chinese medicine theory is beneficial for improving clinical effectiveness. All the RCTs reported that the effectiveness of the treatment intervention based on this theory was better than the outcome in the control group.[11]

One recent study tried to bridge the gap between these Eastern medicine concepts and Western nutritional science. It analyzed the relationship between food composition and its cold or hot properties by looking at 179 different foods. Scientists evaluated the fat, carbohydrate, fiber, water, vitamin, and mineral content of the foods to see if there was any correlation with the categories of hot, cold, or neutral. They even came up with a complex mathematical formula to predict whether a food was warming, cooling, or neutral depending on its chemical composition.[12] Other studies have had similar findings, determining that dietary fiber, magnesium, and copper content are related to the cold nature of foods. Water, proteins, fats, carbohydrates, iron, selenium, and zinc contribute to the hot nature of foods.[13]

Learning about the energetics of foods can help us pick the diet that will best suit us, going a step further than considering just their macros and micronutrient content. This is the secret sauce that I add to all of my patients' treatment plans. Instead of telling them what to eat, I find it's best they learn about their digestive fire, metabolism, and constitution so that they can match these with the right foods. Let's discuss how you can begin to do that for yourself.

Find the Right Fuel for Your Fire

Most imbalances occur when we make wrong food choices that don't match our body's constitution. We put the wrong type of fuel in our body, which compromises the function of our digestive fire. This can lead to all sorts of symptoms and diseases that I regularly see in my practice. These often arise from inflammation, poor circulation, weak digestion, or sluggish metabolism. Hence the saying in Ayurveda that *when the diet is wrong, medicine is of no use, and when the diet is correct, medicine is of no need.*

For example, when we eat foods that match our constitution, they nourish us, boost our metabolism, and increase energy. In contrast, mismatched foods or ones that are highly processed and devoid of nutrients end up draining our energy.

Yes, we're told that foods like avocados, yogurt, nuts, and salads are healthy. However, I have many patients whose bodies just don't work well when they eat these foods. It isn't that they're allergic to them; it's just that the foods don't suit their constitution.

Of course, it's helpful to know what types of foods are hot, cold, damp, or dry, which we'll review in the next sections. But I also teach my patients how to look for signs of excess heat, cold, dryness, or dampness in their body after eating certain foods. Once they can identify these signs of imbalance, they automatically know which foods to eat to balance their yin and yang energies.[14] For instance, salad is healthy, but if you have a "cold" metabolism, eating cold foods like salads might give you gas and leave you feeling unsatisfied. Instead, warm foods such as soups and stews might feel more comforting because the warmth balances out your cold constitution.

Our body and metabolism also constantly change depending on the type of environment where we live and what's going on in our lives. *If everything about us and around us is in a constant state of change, our diet must evolve to keep up.* After all, health is all about striking a balance, so it's important to be aware of outer changes as well.

No matter what life throws at us, we can learn to recognize the shifts in our body and adjust our diet accordingly. When we're deficient in a particular quality, it makes sense to bring the body back into balance by choosing foods that have that quality. Let's review the constitution of foods so you can figure out what your body needs.

Dietary Recommendations for Too Much Heat

Sam falls into this category. From a Western medicine perspective, all his doctors had a hard time treating his symptoms. When I diagnosed him using traditional Chinese medicine, the diagnosis was as clear as day. He suffered from too much heat in the body, which manifests as inflammation. I immediately put him on a diet that would be anti-inflammatory and cooling, along with treating him with herbs and supplements. He didn't realize that healthy foods such as certain nuts and even vegetables like nightshades had contributed to his inflammation.

It took us about six months, but by then, we were able to reduce the medications he had been taking for years. Even his bloodwork showed impressive changes, with inflammation markers at their lowest levels. He was finally relieved of the burning sensation and started to have more regular bowel movements. He not only felt better but also was empowered by gaining a deeper understanding of his symptoms. He continues to use that knowledge every day to stay healthy. The minute he notices signs of imbalance, he adjusts his diet and lifestyle accordingly.

To remedy excess heat, avoid "heating" foods and eat more "cooling" foods.

Think of foods you would normally eat in the summer.

Diet Recommendation for Excess Heat

	Foods to avoid	Eat this instead
Flavors	Spicy, oily, sour excess salt, sugar, chemicals, additives	Sweet, raw, fresh
Preparation method	Fried, smoked, BBQ	Raw salads, smoothies, boiled, steamed, soaked
Spices	Cloves, dry ginger, pepper, mustard	Basil, mint, cardamom, cumin, fennel
Fruits	Sour, citrus, unripe fruits, orange, grapefruit, green apple, berries, lemon, kiwi, pineapple	Ripe fruits such as apple, berries, coconut, date, mango, fig, melons, pomegranate, raisins, prunes, grapes
Vegetables	Garlic, raw onion, tomatoes, chilies, eggplant, horseradish, radish, spinach, beet greens, turnips	Avocado, coconut, cucumber, cauliflower, squash, zucchini, cilantro, celery, artichoke, cooked onions, raw spinach, summer vegetables
Grains	Buckwheat, corn, yeasted bread, rye	Oats, quinoa, sprouted grains, wheat, white rice
Nuts & seeds	All in moderation	Soaked and peeled almonds, pumpkin seeds, flax seeds, and sunflower seeds
Animal protein	Beef, pork, red meat from chicken and turkey, salmon, tuna, saltwater fish, yogurt	White meat from chicken, turkey, freshwater fish, shrimp, buttermilk
Beverages	Very hot teas, coffee, alcohol	Herbal teas such as peppermint, fennel, chamomile

Dietary Recommendations for Too Much Cold

If you have excess cold, the key is to eat foods that are warm, soothing, and easy to digest. Spices and herbs can also help improve digestion. Think of foods that you would typically eat in the winter.

Diet Recommendation for Excess Cold

	Foods to avoid	Eat this instead
Flavors	Sweet	Soft, soupy, warm foods which are easy to digest
Preparation method	Raw salads, smoothies, frozen, iced	Steamed, boiled, roasted, sautéed
Processed foods	Excess salt, sugar, chemicals, additives	Natural foods
Spices	None	Any in moderation can stimulate digestion
Fruits	Unripe fruits	Cooked fruits or ripe fruits such as apple, pear, banana; dried fruits such as prunes, dates, figs
Vegetables	Raw vegetables	Well-cooked vegetables
Grains	Gluten, which can be heavy to digest, soy-based foods such as tofu	Well-cooked grains, sprouted breads (easier to digest)
Nuts & seeds	Limit the amount as they can be hard to digest	Soaked or roasted nuts or nut butters
Animal protein	Ice cream, yogurt, and other dairy products	Well-cooked meat, ideally in a stew
Beverages	Cold or iced beverages	Ginger tea, wine in moderation

Dietary Recommendations for Too Much Dampness

If you have an excess of dampness, you'll benefit from a low-carb and low-fat diet that's high in protein and fiber. Avoiding gluten and dairy can be highly beneficial for decreasing mucus and congestion, while avoiding salty foods can help to relieve fluid retention and edema.

Diet Recommendation for Excess Dampness

	Foods to avoid	Eat this instead
Flavors	Sweet, sour, salty	Pungent, bitter, astringent
Preparation method	Frozen, iced	Roast, bake, grill
Spices	None	Any in moderation can boost metabolism
Fruits	Very sweet or overripe fruits, high calorie fruits such as coconuts, dates, avocados	Astringent fruits such as cranberries, other berries, cherries, pomegranate, lemons
Vegetables	Root and starchy vegetables especially white potatoes	All vegetables especially leafy greens
Grains	Highly processed white flour, white rice	Whole grains that are high in fiber, millets, sprouted breads
Nuts & seeds	Limit the amount as they are high in fat	Seeds over nuts, chia, flax, sunflower, pumpkin seeds
Animal protein	Red meat, saltwater fish, all dairy products	White meat, freshwater fish
Beverages	Cold or iced beverages, drinks high in salt or sugar	Ginger tea, black and green tea

Dietary Recommendations for Too Much Dryness

If you have excess dryness, it's important for you to eat foods that are hydrating and nourishing. Using more water in cooking and eating healthy fats can minimize symptoms associated with dryness. Think of moist foods, with a healthy amount of fat for moisturizing the gut from the inside out.

Diet Recommendation for Excess Dryness

	Foods to avoid	Eat this instead
Flavors/texture	Pungent, bitter, astringent, dry, crunchy, crispy	Sweet, salty, high fat
Preparation method	Roasted, popped, grilled	Steamed, boiled, braised, soups, stews
Spices	Black pepper, chili, horseradish, mustard	All in moderation
Fruits	Astringent fruits such as cranberries, other berries, cherries, pomegranate, lemons	Sweet and juicy such as melons, grapes, citrus
Vegetables	Cruciferous vegetables such as cauliflower, broccoli, brussels sprouts can cause gas	Root and starchy vegetables, avocados, coconut
Grains	Beans, rice cakes, crackers, popcorn	Any grains, mung beans, lentils
Nuts & seeds	None	All preferably as nut butters or nut milks
Animal protein	Red meat	All except red meat
Beverages	Black and green tea	Any herbal, non-caffeinated tea

Eat in Season

A diet should be dynamic and adapt as our body's needs change from time to time and from season to season. Adjusting our diet to match the season is a foreign concept to some people, and many don't know what fruits and vegetables are in season at any given time. If we can buy apples in February and pumpkin in July, how do we keep track? I like to learn what's in season by visiting the local farmers' market. Every week, you'll see a range of different products and get in the habit of eating locally and seasonally.

Our metabolism has evolved to thrive on the food that grows in our surroundings. Just like we adapt to the changing environment around us, so do the plants and animals. Our ancestors didn't have refrigerators and freezers, so they figured out various ways to preserve the foods that were seasonal. This helped them get through periods of limited food availability. Somehow, they managed to survive without blueberries in the winter and sweet potatoes in the summer. If our diet is diverse, we can still get a balanced, nutritious diet in every season.

Another important factor to consider is the nutrient content of fruits and vegetables in different seasons. According to a study performed by the Department of Health and Nutrition Sciences at Montclair State University, the amount of vitamin C in broccoli showed significant seasonal changes. The fall values for vitamin C were almost twice as high as those in spring. Therefore, eating seasonally can also give us more nutrients from the foods we eat.[15]

Visit your local farmers' market on a regular basis to learn more. Please do yourself and the planet a favor by eating local and seasonal foods whenever possible.

What's in Season?

Here's a handy guide from the U.S. Department of Agriculture (USDA) to learn about the main fruits and vegetables found in spring, summer, fall, and winter.[16] Use this list to explore produce that is in season. Depending on where you are, availability might vary a bit based on the temperature and growing conditions.

Spring

Fruits: apple, apricot, banana, kiwi, lime, lemon, pineapple, strawberry, avocado
Vegetables: asparagus, broccoli, cabbage, carrots, celery, collard greens, garlic, herbs, kale, lettuce, mushrooms, onions, peas, radishes, rhubarb, spinach, Swiss chard, turnips

Summer

Fruits: apple, apricot, avocado, banana, blackberry, cantaloupe, cherry, lemon, lime, mango, peach, plum, raspberry, strawberry, watermelon
Vegetables: beet, bell pepper, carrot, celery, corn, cucumber, eggplant, garlic, green beans, herbs, lima beans, okra, summer squash, tomatillo, tomato, zucchini

Fall

Fruits: apple, banana, cranberry, grape, kiwi, lemon, lime, mango, pear, pineapple, raspberry
Vegetables: beet, bell pepper, broccoli, brussels sprouts, cabbage, carrot, cauliflower, celery, collard greens, garlic, ginger, green beans, herbs, kale, lettuce, mushroom, onion, parsnip, pea, potato, pumpkin, radish, rutabaga, spinach, sweet potato, yam, Swiss chard, turnips, winter squash

Winter

Fruits: apple, avocado, banana, grapefruit, kiwi, lemon, lime, orange, pear, pineapple
Vegetables: beet, brussels sprouts, cabbage, carrot, celery, collard greens, herbs, kale, leek, onion, parsnip, potato, pumpkin, rutabaga, sweet potato, yam, Swiss chard, turnips, winter squash

TIPS FOR FINDING THE ROOT CAUSE OF YOUR SYMPTOMS

Trying to find the root cause of symptoms is worth the time and energy. The lessons learned can help you take better care of yourself and prevent future diseases.

- Most diseases occur due to external or internal causes of imbalance.

- External causes are related to the environment around us. From global warming to pollution, we're all susceptible to toxins. They can be the hidden culprit behind many health issues, yet our health-care system doesn't usually address them.

- Internal causes of diseases arise from imbalance in one of the four domains of intentional health: diet, sleep, exercise, and stress management.

- To pick the right diet, it's helpful to discover your constitution: whether you tend to be hot or cold, or damp or dry. Take the quiz to help figure out your constitution. You can also work with an acupuncturist to get a more comprehensive assessment.

- How do you know if your constitution is out of balance? Excess heat, more common in warmer seasons, will manifest as inflammation in different parts of your body. Acne, arthritis, dermatitis, diarrhea with burning sensation in the gut, acid reflux, and overheating are good examples. Excess cold, more common in colder months, will present as cold hands and feet, poor circulation, slow digestion, low energy, and stiff joints. Similarly, dampness is more common in spring or rainy weather, associated with puffy face, swollen ankles, congestion, allergies, more mucus production, and sticky stools. On the other hand, dryness is more common in fall months, leading to dry skin, hair, mouth, and stool; constipation, concentrated urine, and cracking joints.

- Choosing the right foods based on your constitution will help you bring your body back into balance and prevent diseases in the future. For example, if you have symptoms associated with too much heat in the body, it's best to include cooling foods in your diet. Just remember, opposites attract. Refer to the lists above to know which foods and cooking methods will best suit you and help you balance your constitution.

- Take seasons into consideration when you make food choices. Seasonal foods tend to be easier to digest, and they're more likely to match your constitution and metabolism from season to season.

- Print the list of seasonal foods and display it on your refrigerator. The next time you make a grocery list, take a peek at what's in season.

- Make a habit of shopping at your local farmers' market whenever possible. Not only will you get the freshest foods that are in season, but also you'll likely get fewer toxins on your food.

CHAPTER 6

THE ANTI-AGING DETOX

What is the true longevity secret of a yogi who lives for 185 years? Is it a mythical herb, a secret mantra, or the consumption of a superfood? No. There's nothing magical about how yogis turn back the clock, as we explored earlier. Their bodies are no different from ours, and we can do the same . . . *if we pay the detox tax.* When I use the word *detox,* however, I'm not talking about taking a handful of supplements, drinking teas and juices, or getting coffee enemas. It's so much more than that.

In this chapter, I'll introduce toxins and the importance of detoxification, which is a foreign concept in Western culture. In our world, we love the idea of superfoods that are packed with nutrients, but most of the time, it isn't a lack of nutrients that makes us sick. *Most diseases and aging arise from the buildup of toxins in the body, which are byproducts of poor digestion and weak metabolism.*

Of course, we live in an increasingly toxic world. Through the air we breathe, food we eat, water we drink, and everything we touch, we're exposed to thousands of chemicals every day. As toxins build up, we get sicker, and we age more. By detoxing regularly, we can eliminate the poisons and remain youthful.

I had a patient named Lori whose story illustrates the importance of detoxing. She came to me after being diagnosed with fatty liver and high cholesterol. She was hesitant to take the medication for cholesterol since it could affect her liver. (Taking a pill for one condition can sometimes worsen another.) She knew she had to reduce her cholesterol levels because she had a strong family history of heart disease, and she was highly motivated to work on her diet and lifestyle to optimize her health. We decided to try that approach before resorting to medications.

Given the diagnosis of fatty liver and the fact that the liver is our most important detox organ, I suspected sluggishness in her ability to get rid of toxins. Before starting her regimen, she underwent extensive lab testing and imaging so we could gather objective data to track over time. Our goal was to monitor her progress over three months and decide if she still needed the medications. At the end of the chapter, I'll give you an update on how the treatment worked for Lori. But first, let's examine the science of how the body rids itself of toxins.

THE SCIENCE: THE "RHYTHM" OF THE LIVER

Just as there are internal and external causes of diseases that make us sick, there are internal and external causes of toxins that accumulate in our body over time. They get in the way of normal physiological processes, accelerate aging, and eventually lead to illness.

External sources of toxins are the same as those we discussed before. In our modern world, we're exposed to so many chemicals that it comes as no surprise that they often make us sick. They can cause breast, ovarian, and prostate cancer, as well as diabetes, heart disease, obesity, and infertility.[1]

Internal sources of toxins are the result of poor digestion, improper diet, and slow metabolism. These internally generated toxins accumulate in our body over time and lead to several health issues. Common symptoms such as fatigue, sluggishness, aches and pains, inflammation in the skin or joints, and headaches are among those associated with toxicity.

So, how does our body get rid of the muck that piles up over time, clogging our organs? Enter the liver, our main detox organ.

It's a metabolic and detox powerhouse, although it's assisted by our kidneys and gut microbiome.

Pretty much everything that enters our body—food, medications, or toxins—must pass through the liver to be processed. If we want our food to nourish us, medications to work properly, and toxins to be eliminated, we need to pay special attention to it.

But first, we must consider the connection between the liver and the circadian rhythm. We've explored the role our internal clock plays in our health. When it's synchronized with nature, our body works effortlessly. When we're out of sync with our natural cycles, it can become the root cause of many conditions.

The circadian rhythm is controlled by our main internal clock, which is in the brain. However, we also have several important peripheral clocks in the rest of the body, including in the gut, adrenal glands, pancreas, and liver. Disturbances in communication between the main clock and the ones in different organs have been implicated in diseases such as obesity and neuropsychiatric disorder.[2]

The liver is tightly synchronized with the master clock in the brain. It's involved in managing our blood sugar, processing fat and protein from our food, and even activating hormones like the thyroid. If our liver clock is out of sync, it can affect conditions like diabetes, high cholesterol, fatty liver, and thyroid issues.

Our liver performs different functions depending on what we're doing from moment to moment and based on temperature and seasonal changes. For example, when we're sleeping and fasting, the liver will focus more on detoxification. When we're active, eating, or digesting, it will focus more on our metabolism and processing nutrients.[3]

According to Eastern medicine, the liver also has different daytime and nighttime functions. During the day, it helps process the food we eat, so anything that affects our daily routine will have an impact on how well our liver is able to do its job.

While we've talked about our digestive fire and how to eat the right foods to match our constitution, which engages the liver in the daytime, we haven't yet discussed the liver's nighttime function: detoxing. First, the liver turns toxic compounds into inert, water-soluble substances that can be eliminated from the body. Once it completes this task, the waste is then handed over to the gut and the kidneys. As we discussed in the gut microbiome chapter, the army of tiny bacteria plays a vital role in this detox process. Good bacteria work with the liver to further process toxins. Bad bacteria, on the other hand, can undo the work of the liver and send the toxins back into circulation. Besides the conditions listed, a buildup of toxins has been linked to obesity and the dysregulation of our immune and reproductive systems.[4]

As I mentioned, our kidneys are also part of the detoxification team. Most of us think of them as simply organs that make urine, but they're responsible for many important functions, such as maintaining the amount of fluid in the body, balancing electrolytes, regulating blood pressure, and even activating vitamin D. They play a particularly important role in eliminating drugs from the body. If the kidneys aren't functioning properly, it can affect drug metabolism and potentially cause toxicity.[5]

Unfortunately, our detox organs rarely get any love from us. Instead, we worry about our cardiovascular health, so we exercise. We go on a diet to improve our metabolic health and control our weight. Even when we learn about the importance of these organs, we still aren't sure how to take better care of them.

This is where the wisdom of Eastern medicine can guide us. According to Ayurveda, our metabolism has two functions: metabolizing food and detoxification. There's a time, place, and process for each of these jobs. During the day, our body focuses on processing the food we eat, so it's active metabolically. At night, instead of digestion, it focuses on cleanup, repair, regeneration, and taking out the garbage. We can't do both at the same time efficiently. We may love the idea of multitasking, but our body works best when we dedicate time and effort to one of these functions or the other.

Yes, our body is an astonishing piece of machinery, but even machines have to be cleaned, maintained, and fixed at times. Fortunately, our body knows exactly how to take care of itself. It has ingrained knowledge of how to nourish, repair, and rejuvenate. But if our body is so capable, why do we age and get sick? Let's delve deeper into the answer to that question.

WHAT GOES WRONG?

We live in a world that's always on the go. We rarely give our bodies a break or breathing room to repair and rejuvenate. We expect them to work around the clock. You already know that the constant disruption of our circadian rhythm affects our metabolism during the day. It also affects our ability to heal and detox at night.

Our metabolism's two main functions have specific names: anabolism (buildup) and catabolism (breakdown). During the day, it's in the catabolic state, in which it's busy breaking down food to generate energy. We use this energy to help us power through our daily activities. However, burning calories leads to the production of free radicals, which can cause damage to our cells and lead to wear and tear over time.

At night, our metabolism shifts gears, diverting its attention to anabolic activities. These include clearing out toxins, repairing cell damage that occurred during the catabolic phase, and rebuilding cells.[6]

This complex process is regulated by many players, but two main hormones play a particularly vital role: *growth hormone* and *cortisol*. Considered an anabolic hormone, growth hormone helps build tissue. Even in adults, it's crucial for building muscle, bone, and brain cells, along with reducing belly fat and increasing the ratio of good to bad cholesterol.[7] That sounds like the fountain of youth to me. No wonder it's often used by athletes to boost their performance and sometimes touted as an elixir to reverse aging.

Most of the growth hormone in adults is released in the first 90 minutes or so of sleep between 10 p.m. and midnight.

If we go to bed late, we miss out on the growth hormone surge.[8]

Even if we sleep in to catch up, the amount of growth hormone we release isn't enough to make up for a later bedtime.

On the other hand, we have the master catabolic hormone, cortisol, that takes care of our circadian rhythm and metabolism while the sun is shining. Cortisol has many functions in the human body, such as mediating the stress response and regulating metabolism, the inflammatory response, and immune function.[9] Its levels peak later in our sleep toward early morning to get us ready for the day.

Of course, some wear and tear of our cells and organs is expected as a byproduct of our metabolism. As our body uses up energy, it produces something called *oxidative stress* on the cells, which leads to aging over time.[10] This is why it's important to allow for adequate time at night to fix the wear and tear as much as possible by removing the toxins caused by daytime metabolic activities.

A balance between these two hormones is key to maintaining our overall health. Our diet and lifestyle choices play a pivotal role in this process. Let's examine how our lack of routine may cause some of the most common symptoms of poor detoxification.

Common Symptom/Condition #1: Improper Sleep and Accelerated Aging

You probably didn't expect to read about sleep in a chapter on detoxification, but it's actually a vital component of the process. Unfortunately, we often take sleep for granted and sacrifice it in the name of our modern lifestyle. It can be a nuisance, sometimes getting in the way of our work and play. Whether we must burn the midnight oil to study, get work done, or just have a good time with friends, sleep is often deemed less important. We try to make up the loss by loading up on caffeine the next day or "catching up" on sleep over the weekend, but you already know how this type of irregular sleep pattern can lead to chronic disruption of our circadian rhythm.

We tend to appreciate sleep only when it eludes us. Then we'll do anything to simply obtain a few hours of restful shut-eye. In prior chapters, we saw how our irregular routine, exposure to blue light, and high stress levels can all affect our sleep. We might think we shouldn't care as long as we can get through our day seemingly unaffected, with the help of a little caffeine. But studies have shown that the amount of energy our body spends during sleep is reduced to two-thirds of the amount when we're awake. This conserved energy is redirected to regenerative, adaptive, and anabolic processes such as cellular repair, immune function, and organizing neural networks in the brain.[11] Regardless of the reduction in energy expended, all these tasks set the stage for quite a busy night shift.

Many studies have also demonstrated that poor sleep accelerates aging. For example, it affects our telomeres, which are DNA protein structures that act as caps to protect and stabilize the ends of our chromosomes. They're a marker of cellular aging, as the length of our telomeres declines with age. Shorter telomere length has been associated with cardiovascular disease, strokes, diabetes, cancer, depression, chronic stress, and premature death. We want our telomeres to be long and healthy so that they can protect our DNA, keep the wrinkles away, and help prevent us from developing many of the chronic diseases that accompany aging.

A recent study evaluated more than five thousand older adults to see if there was an association between quality of sleep and telomere length. The participants were asked about their sleep quality. Overall, 16 percent reported never feeling well rested in the morning; 25.7 percent always woke up during the night, and 12.8 percent always woke up too early in the morning. Those who never felt rested upon rising had significantly shorter telomere lengths than those who always felt rested in the morning.[12]

One of the questions I always ask my patients is whether they feel rested when they wake up. Indirectly, I'm trying to get an idea of what their telomeres look like.

Often, we focus on the duration of sleep. We're told to get our daily dose of eight hours, but the quality of the sleep matters as well. If our eight hours in bed are spent tossing and turning, snoring, waking up frequently to urinate, or worrying about the next day, they aren't providing the kind of sleep we need to properly detoxify.

Common Symptom/Condition #2: Brain Fog, Forgetfulness, and Alzheimer's Disease

Just like the rest of the body, the brain also shifts its attention to detox and repair at night. There are significant changes in the electrical activity, blood flow, and cerebrospinal fluid movement when we're in deep sleep. The cerebrospinal fluid that surrounds the brain helps flush out metabolic waste from the area. When we're sleeping, the metabolic activity and the blood flow to the brain goes down. This allows for extra space for the fluid to move in and clear out the toxins that have accumulated throughout the day.[13]

This finding has major implications for research related to neurodegenerative conditions such as Alzheimer's disease, which are thought to be caused by a buildup of toxic proteins. Very soon, we might have a diagnostic test to measure the flow of the cerebrospinal fluid in a variety of neurological conditions. Researchers are also looking at how electromagnetic stimulation of brain waves can be used as a treatment.[14]

Whether or not we ever develop Alzheimer's disease, we have all experienced the downside of sleep deprivation in our lives, whether it's making a small and inconvenient mistake such as forgetting our wallet at home or having a more serious event like a motor vehicle accident. Our brain cells take their sweet time becoming operational when they haven't received adequate rest overnight. A few nights of revelry aren't going to cause major health issues, but prolonged sleep disruption can have a lasting impact on our brain health.

Dr. David Dinges, one of the top sleep researchers, and other scientists have shown that cognitive performance and vigilant attention begin to decline quickly after we stay awake more than 16 hours. Plus, sleep deficits from partial sleep deprivation can accumulate over time. Even shortchanging ourselves of an hour of sleep just to scroll through social media has a cumulative effect on our health.

Dr. Dinges and his colleagues developed the psychomotor vigilance test (PVT), a simple neurocognitive test to assess an individual's ability to sustain attention and respond to signals in a timely manner. It has reliably detected the effects of disrupted or fragmented sleep and has also shown that the timing of the sleep matters. A growing body of evidence suggests that the continuity and timing of sleep may be as important as the total amount of time spent sleeping.[15]

Besides forgetfulness and sluggishness, lack of sleep can also impact our mood. One-third of U.S. adults report sleeping less than the recommended amount, and approximately 20 percent live with a mental illness. It comes as no surprise that there's a connection between how well our brains rest at night and our mental well-being. A large cross-sectional study looking at more than 270,000 adults found that 13 percent of the participants experienced inadequate sleep, and 14.1 percent experienced frequent mental distress. Participants who averaged six hours or less of sleep per night were about two and a half times more likely to have frequent mental distress than those who slept more than six hours.[16]

It's important to remember that as we snooze, our brain is busy with memory processing, detox, and hormonal shifts, all in an effort to repair and rejuvenate. If all goes well, we wake up well rested and refreshed for the day ahead. If not, it can be significantly detrimental to our entire body over time.

Common Symptom/Condition #3: Fatty Liver

Fatty liver is a condition that's been on the rise, although many people haven't heard of it. It can be caused by alcohol intake, but what I'm talking about here is nonalcoholic fatty liver disease (NAFLD). According to the National Institutes of Health, about 24 percent of U.S. adults have NAFLD, and it's becoming one of the top causes of liver disease.[17]

Multiple factors are involved in the complex development of this condition, such as obesity, fat toxicity, inflammation, imbalanced dietary intake, low physical activity, the gut microbiome, and socioeconomic aspects, along with genetic predisposition. The latest research has added another important risk factor to the list: sleep disruption. Since the master clock in our brain is synchronized with the liver, any disruption in the circadian rhythm, including sleep disruption, will affect the function of this important organ. Problems with the liver may in turn affect sleep patterns. Sleep should be added to the list of modifiable behaviors to optimize our liver's ability to perform its detoxification functions and also prevent or manage NAFLD.

When I see patients with fatty liver, I always inquire about their sleep patterns. This surprises them since they expect me to focus on changing their diet and exercise habits to lose weight. They're often told that if they just lost weight, their fatty liver would improve. While that's true, if sleep isn't optimized, a better diet and exercise can only achieve so much.

In many people, sleep disruption is even the root cause of fatty liver, because it directly affects their ability to detox. Studies have shown that night-shift workers[18] and people who work long hours[19] are more likely to develop NAFLD. As with anything else, I have to get to the root cause to treat fatty liver. A detailed sleep assessment and a strategy to optimize sleep quality will make a significant difference, along with proper diet and exercise.

Common Symptom/Condition #4: Aging Muscles

As we grow older, our organs tend to take a beating, but we aren't usually as aware of these changes as we are of the wrinkles on our forehead. But another frustrating visible sign of aging is loss of muscle tone. Who wouldn't want to walk around with a six-pack and toned biceps regardless of their age? But suddenly, exercise doesn't have the same effect on our muscles as it once did.

Since muscle literally does the heavy lifting for us, it's a metabolically active organ. During the day when we're active, our muscles use up a lot of energy. As with every organ and cell, burning calories and working all day long can bring undue wear and tear to our beloved muscles. If we want them to perform well, they also need a break and tune-up every night.

Our anabolic hero, growth hormone, helps us remain fit and toned by increasing lean muscle mass and reducing body fat. Unfortunately, with age, there's a decline of about 14 percent of lean muscle mass per decade of life, beginning in the second decade. Wouldn't it be nice if we could simply supplement with growth hormone as we get older? While studies have demonstrated that supplementation can help in people with a deficiency or in older adults, that doesn't give us the full picture.[20]

It's the yin-and-yang synchrony between growth hormone at night and cortisol during the day that's key to optimal muscle health. Again, it's the dance between our body clocks and detoxification processes.

Very often, a decrease in muscle mass occurs not only because of age-related changes in growth hormone but also due to chronic sleep loss, which tilts the balance toward the catabolic effect of cortisol. In this case, instead of making and repairing muscle at night, we end up with more wear and tear.

The effects of even one night of sleep loss on our muscles can be significant. One study evaluated young adults who were subjected to one night of total sleep deprivation. They experienced an 18 percent reduction in muscle protein synthesis, a 21 percent increase in cortisol, and a 24 percent decrease in testosterone. The authors of the study concluded that a single night of total sleep deprivation can be a precursor to the kinds of changes in body composition that come with chronic sleep deprivation.[21]

Most of us aren't training to run a marathon or play in the Super Bowl, but the business of muscle recovery and sleep is especially relevant for athletes and military personnel. Research shows they're particularly susceptible to the deleterious effects of sleep deprivation on muscle tissue. Sleep optimization can potentially help the recovery from exercise-induced muscle injuries through increasing growth hormone and controlling local inflammation.[22]

Whether you're a weekend warrior or an athlete, an optimal amount of rest is key for muscle recovery. If you want to lose stubborn belly fat and improve your muscle tone, look closely at the balance between growth hormone and cortisol. Your sleep is the link between the two.

Now let's turn our attention to the best ways you can make sure your body consistently rejuvenates and takes out the garbage so that you can stay as healthy and youthful as possible.

THE SOLUTION: MAINTAIN YOUR BODY AND DETOX REGULARLY

When we buy a new car, how long it lasts will depend on its current condition and how well we maintain it. Often, we're inclined to spend a fortune on the latest model with all the bells and whistles. Yet, in a few years, we encounter issues that require our attention. Whether we have a new luxury car or a 20-year-old model, these machines are prone to wear and tear. We can have routine oil changes, pay attention to every check-engine light, and follow the instructions of our mechanic. Or we can wait until something goes wrong, leaving us stranded on the side of the road.

The same is true for our health. Some of us are born with a body that runs like a Lamborghini, while others are working with a lemon. Not everyone can win the genetic lottery, but genetics are still only a small part of the equation. How well we tend to our body and maintain it will ultimately determine its longevity. Even if we have a genetic predisposition to certain diseases, we can overcome it with the right diet and lifestyle choices. Our health destiny is indeed often in our hands.

Unlike Eastern medicine's focus on prevention, Western medicine tends to emphasize only the cure—once a disease has already taken hold. Therefore, the concept of detox is so important. It's all about preventing disease and eliminating the root cause before it has an opportunity to create further—and possibly irreversible—harm.

If we want to remain healthy and slow down aging, it's key to maintain our bodies and detox on a regular basis.

Just like an engine needs an oil change, a cleaning, and a tune-up from time to time, so do we. For example, we regularly put gas in the car or get a car wash to keep it clean and running. Every few months, we get rid of the accumulated sludge that we can't see since it's deep in the engine. Our body accumulates sludge as well, and it slows us down. Simply eating a healthy meal, running on a treadmill, and taking care of our outward appearance isn't enough. We also need to take steps daily to maintain our body, as well as conduct a deeper detox from time to time to eliminate hidden gunk. Toxins, whether external from our environment or internal from poor digestion, need to be removed in a timely manner before they age us prematurely and create disease. Besides optimizing your sleep, let's review what you can do to promote healthy detox and enhance repair and rejuvenation.

Utilize Intermittent Fasting

Many of my patients have tried intermittent fasting, but there's a right way and a wrong way to do it. Let's explore the right way.

First of all, stop and think about how it was for our ancestors. It wasn't until about a hundred years ago that we started having easier access to food thanks to better methods of preserving and transporting food. Eating three meals a day was never the norm and was reserved only for royalty. Even to this day, access to three meals isn't a reality for more than a billion people on the planet. Rewinding back further to our hunter-gatherer days, we were lucky to get two meals a day most of the time. It was more common to go hungry, since access to food wasn't always guaranteed. Fasting, not feasting, is what our body evolved to handle.

Nowadays, with a plethora of food options, we're made to believe that we should eat three meals per day and have a couple of snacks in between to properly fuel our bodies. If that was always the case, how did our ancestors survive? We don't usually get sick in the Western world from missing a vitamin or nutrient.

Instead, I see people suffering from eating more than what their body can digest. Most diseases in our world arise from an accumulation of toxins as a product of poor metabolism and inadequate detoxification. Eliminating toxins is just as important as getting the right nutrients.

When most people consider the idea of dieting or fasting, however, they think it's about cutting their total calories. I try to educate and empower my patients to get out of the calorie mindset. It's indeed eye-opening when they realize that how their body processes food depends on what time they eat.

A key lesson my patients learn is that late-night eating is one of the worst things they can do for their metabolism. Even if it's a "healthy" meal, eating later interferes with the detox process and adversely affects the metabolism. It also causes much bigger glucose and insulin spikes and even affects sleep. When people wake up the next morning, their fasting blood sugar tends to be higher, and they feel more sluggish overall. I even place some of my patients on continuous glucose monitors to give them an insight as to how their blood sugar spikes in response to different foods at different times. Once they see how their metabolism works, it's much easier to personalize their diet.

Research conducted at the University of Pennsylvania supports the finding that late-night eating is detrimental to our health. In this study, a group of healthy-weight adults underwent two conditions for eight weeks. During the first eight-week period, they ate meals between 8 A.M. and 7 P.M. Then they skipped two weeks and spent another eight weeks eating a delayed diet from 12 P.M. to 11 P.M. Sleep was constant during both periods from 11 P.M. to 9 A.M. The researchers found that compared to eating earlier in the day, prolonged delayed eating increased weight, insulin, and cholesterol levels. It also negatively affected fat metabolism and hormonal markers implicated in heart disease, diabetes, and other health problems.[23] There was no difference in the number of calories they ate in the two eight-week periods; it was just about the timing of their meals.

I recommend to my patients that they restrict their eating window to 8 to 10 hours and allow for a fasting window of 14 to 16 hours. It seems daunting at first, but it's absolutely doable and sustainable. Most people think that by skipping breakfast and lunch, they're getting in their fasting hours and cutting calories. What ends up happening, however, is that their dinner then becomes their biggest meal. Instead of detoxing at night, their poor liver is still working on their dinner. This can wreak havoc on their metabolic health.

The right way to do intermittent fasting is to use sunrise and sunset as your reference point (unless, of course, you live in a place with the midnight sun). For most of us, we can use 7 A.M. and 7 P.M. as a reasonable estimate for sunrise and sunset. *I advise my patients to eat their first meal within three hours of waking up and their last meal of the day at least three hours before bedtime.* Lunch should be their biggest meal, and they should opt for a lighter, low-carb dinner to prevent late-night insulin spikes.

This approach also works for weight loss. While most people are advised to simply cut calories, restricting our eating window can give us the same results.[24] This is because, on average, people naturally reduce their caloric consumption by approximately 20 percent when they stick to an eating window.[25] There's no need to torture ourselves with counting calories.

If you need more reasons to put this plan into action, we know that restricting the eating window can help reduce body weight, improve glucose tolerance, protect from fatty liver, increase metabolic flexibility, reduce cholesterol and blood pressure, and improve gut function and cardiometabolic health.[26]

How long after changing your eating pattern will you see results if you've always skipped breakfast and eaten dinner at 9 P.M.? Studies have shown that just four days of eating most of your foods in the earlier window from 8 A.M. to 2 P.M. will lead to reduced levels of the hunger hormone ghrelin, decreased desire to eat, and an increase in fat burning.[27]

Intermittent fasting allows for the body to dedicate enough time for detox, repair, and regeneration. Then, when you do eat during the day, you digest the food better and create fewer toxins. It's a win-win situation.

Detoxing Heavy Metals

To get an idea of how well your body can detox if it isn't digesting food all day, let me give you an example. In one study, participants were asked to fast for 10 days to see what impact it would have on heavy metal levels in their body. During the 10 days, the subjects received 250 milliliters of organic juice at midday, 20 grams of honey, and 250 milliliters of vegetable soup in the evening, leading to a daily calorie intake of about 250. They were recommended to drink at least two to three liters of water or noncaloric, organic herbal teas. The reintroduction of food occurred in steps from 800 to 1,600 calories per day, consisting of an organic, vegetarian diet.

After 10 days, their urinary arsenic dropped by 72 percent, nickel by 15 percent, and lead by 30 percent. Surprisingly, fatigue, sleep disorders, headaches, and hunger were reduced.[28] This type of fast should be done only under close medical supervision.

Pay Attention to Elimination

The concept of metabolism, detox, and elimination can be a bit confusing. When I discuss them with my patients, I use a simple analogy. Let's say you're hosting a party. You've been busy all day in the kitchen, preparing the food—this is like your metabolism during the day. As a byproduct of your cooking, there will be a mess to clean up. Your guests leave, and then comes the night shift—cleaning duty. Just like your liver works hard to detox at night, you try to clean up as best you can. You put away the clean dishes and put the trash in garbage bags.

Exhausted from all the chores, you head to bed for a good night's rest. You wake up in the morning and realize you forgot to take out the trash. As clean as your house may be, it still stinks!

> Detox is cleaning the house, and elimination is taking out the trash.

How exactly do toxins leave our body? Simply put, if we want anything to leave, we must poop, pee, or sweat it out. In Western medicine, we place a lot of emphasis on what we put into our body but hardly pay any attention to what comes out the other end. Remember what I said about being able to tell a lot about someone's health by their poop? Questions about your bowel movements, the color of your urine, and the smell of your sweat can yield valuable information. Let's talk about all three.

Bowel Movements

How many bowel movements should we have? The official answer is that anywhere from three bowel movements per day to three per week is considered normal. In my opinion, however, depending on your fiber intake, normal consists of one to two well-formed bowel movements per day that are yellow to brown in color.

Unfortunately, I've had patients who thought one bowel movement a week was normal, while others thought five per *day* was normal. We don't talk about it enough, so most people have no clue. Doctors usually address it only if someone complains of constipation or diarrhea.

Yet, more than four million Americans have frequent constipation, which accounts for 2.5 million physician visits a year, according to the National Digestive Diseases Information Clearinghouse. We are indeed a constipated nation. Recent studies indicate that chronic constipation can cause serious long-term effects on our health. It can increase the risk of colorectal cancer, and the risk increases with the severity of the constipation.[29] It can significantly increase the risk of Parkinson's disease in men,[30] and an analysis of more than 70,000 postmenopausal women found that constipation is a marker for heart disease.[31]

Common sense would dictate that we should eliminate the waste from our body at least once a day. The longer it sticks around, the more likely it will cause problems. Even ancient Egyptians believed that decomposing waste can poison the body.[32] Eastern medicine places significant emphasis on optimizing bowel movements for treatment, prevention, and detoxification.[33]

To regulate your bowel movements, try these three steps:

1. ***Increase the amount of fiber in your diet.*** It's the supernutrient that can protect you from cancer, keep your gut microbiome happy, maintain your waistline, and reduce your risk of diabetes and heart disease.[34] Since there are many different types of fiber, I recommend getting at least 30 grams daily from a variety of sources: fruits, vegetables, legumes, and whole grains. Each has its unique role, just like vitamins. Take a fiber supplement, if necessary.

2. ***Drink a big glass of warm water first thing in the morning on an empty stomach.*** This stimulates your gastrocolic reflex, which is your stomach's way of telling your colon to get things going. In Ayurvedic and Chinese medicine, warm water is your gut's best friend.

3. ***Squat!*** Yes, I said *squat*. People in the parts of the world that use squatting toilets in the floor experience fewer hemorrhoids. We have evolved to poop in the forest while squatting down, not sitting on porcelain thrones. One of the reasons why some people have a hard time passing a bowel movement and suffering from hemorrhoids is because of their anatomy. When we squat, it relaxes certain muscles in our pelvic floor that allows for a smoother passage of stool. When we sit instead, we often must strain to overcome this hurdle, which can eventually lead to hemorrhoids. A simple solution is to use a stool that's about six inches high. The goal is to get your knees close to your chest, which will relax the right muscles in your pelvic floor.

These modifications can reduce straining, empty your bowels better, and reduce the time you spend on the toilet.[35]

Proper Urination

I'm surprised that so many people barely glance at what comes out of their bodies in the toilet. I always encourage my patients to look before they flush, as it's a daily health report.

When I discuss urination, my patients often ask me how much water they should be drinking. According to the U.S. National Academies of Sciences, Engineering, and Medicine, the recommended amount of daily fluid intake is about 15 and a half cups per day for men and 11 and a half cups per day for women. I wish the answer were that simple, however. Everyone has a different metabolic and physiologic requirement for water. One way to know how much you should drink is by paying attention to how much urine you produce.

When someone is very sick and admitted to the hospital, this is how we keep track of their kidney function. We track how much fluid they take in and how much urine they produce. For most of us, a rough estimate will suffice. If you're urinating every two to three hours, and the color of your urine is clear to light yellow, you're doing a good job at keeping yourself hydrated. If your urine is always concentrated despite drinking a lot of water, if the color is more amber or reddish brown, if it has an odor, or if it's very frothy, you should consult your doctor.

Before modern advances in medicine, urine was used to detect all sorts of diseases. Its color, frequency, smell, quantity, and ease of passage were closely evaluated. Diabetes was detected either through a sweet taste of the urine or the fact that ants were attracted to it due to its high sugar content.[36] Fortunately, we don't have to go through the taste test anymore. A simple glance before you flush is good enough.

Sweating

From ancient times in cultures like the Mayan, Greek, Roman, and Turkish, bathhouses were social epicenters for the health benefits of steam-room therapy. Even in the present day, some countries, like those in Scandinavia, have continued the tradition with sauna as part of their lifestyle.

Most of us come across saunas at spas or gyms. We might partake occasionally for their relaxing effect, but some people don't consider sitting in a hot box and breaking into a sweat to be particularly calming. Nevertheless, sweating can potentially help eliminate certain toxins. Heavy metals such as arsenic, lead, mercury, and cadmium can be found in higher levels in our sweat than in our blood or urine.[37] While we need more research to evaluate the detoxifying effects of sauna therapy, it makes sense that sweating would be beneficial to us.

In Eastern medicine, it's used not only for potential detox benefits but also for overall health. It can reduce blood pressure, improve cardiac function in patients with heart failure, improve lung function in patients with asthma and chronic bronchitis, reduce pain, and improve mobility in patients with rheumatic disease.[38] A large study conducted in Finland found that regular sauna bathing significantly reduced cardiovascular risk and mortality.[39] The researchers even saw a reduction in dementia and Alzheimer's disease risk. People who used a sauna four to seven times weekly saw the most impressive benefits.[40]

A traditional Finnish sauna uses dry heat with an average temperature of 113 to 220 degrees Fahrenheit. Humidity is generally low—between 10 to 20 percent—and can be adjusted by throwing water on hot rocks. Most people spend an average of 5 to 20 minutes in the sauna, often alternating between its heat and a cold shower. We can lose about a pound of sweat in one session. So, of course, hydration is extremely important.

If you can't tolerate the high temperatures in a typical sauna, another option is a far-infrared sauna that uses infrared waves. These waves heat up your internal core temperature without the need to heat up a whole room. The temperature is more tolerable at 120 to 140 degrees Fahrenheit.

Breaking a sweat mimics cardiovascular exercise like walking or jogging. The heat causes your blood vessels to dilate, and your heart rate and heart-pumping function ramp up. It also affects your autonomic nervous system, which controls temperature regulation. Since several toxins and heavy metal levels are higher in our sweat, regular sweating through sauna therapy can help you eliminate them on a regular basis. And if you don't have access to a sauna, you can break a sweat through regular exercise.

One word of caution before you don your bathing suit: Since sauna therapy mimics exercise and puts your heart to work, it's best avoided if you have a significant heart condition. Discuss it with your physician first.

Regardless of your overall health, don't forget to drink plenty of fluids before and after your sauna session, and monitor your urine output to make sure you're getting enough water.

These steps can all have a huge impact on your health. In the beginning of the chapter, I mentioned my patient Lori. We used these strategies to help her feel better. To jump-start her health journey, I created a customized detox plan that involved optimizing sleep, intermittent fasting, a daily routine, and an exercise regimen. She suffered from occasional constipation, so I prescribed herbs that would help her have a daily bowel movement.

We also cleaned up her diet and lifestyle to be mindful of her exposure to chemicals through foods, water, household products, and even cosmetics. None of these steps involved drastic changes, and they were done gradually in a way that she could maintain for years to come.

It took a few weeks for Lori to adjust to her new routine. She was able to stick to it because she felt so much better. She no longer woke up feeling groggy and relying on coffee to get through the day. She was more mindful of what and when she ate. She made her mealtimes and bedtimes a priority. By educating herself about the hidden chemicals that were affecting her health, she felt more confident about her choices. Her liver, kidneys, and gut microbiome were delighted to see a reduced toxic load.

Just a few months later, her repeat bloodwork showed that her abnormal liver function and cholesterol had both returned to normal and there was no longer a need for medications. We also repeated her liver ultrasound, which no longer showed evidence of fatty liver. Her hard work and dedication had paid off! I was delighted to take the diagnosis of fatty liver off her chart.

TIPS TO HELP YOUR BODY DETOX

Detoxing is not something we "do" with diets, herbs, or supplements. Our body knows exactly how to do it daily. It's just that our lifestyle often gets in the way. Follow these steps to keep your body's detox efforts functioning well:

- Routine is so important when it comes to supporting detoxification, repair, and rejuvenation. Besides your circadian rhythm, regular bedtime and mealtimes will keep your liver clock synchronized.

- The time that you go to bed and the quality of your sleep are just as important as how many hours you sleep. The goal is to optimize your sleep during the early hours of the night, when growth hormone is hard at work.

- I find the intermittent fasting window of a minimum of 12 hours and a maximum of 16 hours easy to implement. The key is avoiding late, heavy dinners so that your body can focus on detoxing at night instead of digestion.

- Don't forget to take out the garbage. Daily bowel movements ensure that you have a happy, healthy gut and a balanced gut microbiome (another detox powerhouse besides the liver).

- Always look before you flush. Keep an eye out for how many times you urinate and what your urine looks like. Adjust your fluid intake accordingly.

- Breaking a sweat is good for you for many reasons. Whether you do it with a brisk walk or in a sauna, add it to your detox checklist.

CHAPTER 7

THE MIND-BODY CONNECTION

Even though my parents practiced yoga and meditation on a regular basis, I couldn't be bothered with those kinds of things during my teen years. Then at the age of 21, after deciding to take a year off to explore the world before starting medical school, I found myself in India, visiting relatives. I had worked for a few months to make enough to finance my adventure on my own dime.

Once I was in India, my uncle suggested I attend a 10-day meditation retreat in a nearby town, since I wouldn't have another chance after medical school started. I had six months at my disposal, so 10 days didn't sound like a lot.

Of course, this was before it was commonplace to search everything on the Internet. With nothing but basic information, I packed my bag. It was a rough bus ride out to the rural area, where I was dropped off on the side of the road and made my way to the retreat. At the center, I was instructed to hand over all my valuables. These included my wallet, books, and iPod. All I could keep were my clothes and toiletries. I also learned for the first time that it would be a silent retreat.

This was pre-iPhone, TikTok, Instagram, and Twitter, so I wasn't addicted to my Nokia brick phone. Still, going 10 days without speaking to anyone, reading a book, or listening to music was more than a typical American 21-year-old was prepared for.

I thought the hardest part would be waking up at 4 A.M. and not being able to speak. But there was something else that made me look for the Exit sign. Since a full belly isn't ideal for meditation, our meals were limited to a light breakfast, healthy lunch, and a snack in the evening. The detox of the mind was indeed tied to the detox of the body, so our diet and lifestyle had to be in sync.

The first few days, I found it unbearable to sit cross-legged on a cushion, meditating at 4 A.M. Then came the stomach growls and mind-numbing pain in my legs that started to fall asleep faster than the rest of me. I was the youngest one in our group of 18 people, yet I had the hardest time sitting on the floor. They had chairs available for people with bad knees or hips, but I was unwilling to give up my youthful pride. Instead, I followed the mantra that we were taught: "This, too, shall pass." I had heard that phrase many times, and it sounded like good advice. But try practicing it in real life while you feel numb from the waist down and you're trying to focus on your breath while distracted by hunger pangs. Nothing about the experience was "passing" quickly enough.

I'm not exaggerating when I say that by day three, I had conjured up my step-by-step escape from the center, mostly inspired by the movie *The Rock*. The meditation center was my Alcatraz. I would simply have to hitchhike or climb on top of the bus and make my way home to my relatives in the city. Of course, I had no money or phone, and the safety of hitchhiking or riding on top of a bus was a questionable detail. But all I wanted was to sleep in, eat a feast, scream at the top of my lungs, and listen to some heavy metal music. Never mind that I wouldn't normally do any of those things.

Then something interesting happened on day four. I woke up on my own at 4 A.M., and I wasn't ravenous. Even when meditating, I stopped thinking about food and found it easier to sit still in the posture. Over the next few days, a sense of calm and ease enveloped me. All the events that had been playing in my head slowed down. My senses became sharper. It was almost like I had put on glasses and could see things around me that I'd never noticed or like my ears had popped after a long flight. I could hear the birds and the bees that had been lost to my awareness before.

While meditating, I could feel my heartbeat and appreciate how it synchronized with my breathing. The slightest movement in my body would alter my breathing and, in turn, my heartbeat. With my mind and senses no longer pulled in different directions, I felt lighter on my feet, in my heart, and in my mind. *Once our brain settles down, the true nature of our mind is revealed to us.*

Most of us spend years chasing the noise and distractions of our lives, preventing our body and mind from manifesting their true nature. Our Alcatraz is of our own making, and we carry it with us everywhere we go.

Each day after day four of my meditation retreat brought me more serenity and joy, a feeling of home, and being present in the moment with all my senses, my mind, and my body. It was quite a transformation in just 10 days. All I had to do was *less* of everything we do every day. Less was indeed more in this case. When I looked at my face in the mirror properly for the first time after leaving the retreat, I was shocked. There was an effervescent glow on my skin, and the whites of my eyes were the whitest I'd ever seen. I felt radiant inside out.

I wished that sense of peace and joy could last forever. Such magic starts to fade as we step out into the world. Still, the transformation that occurred in my mind and body in India had a lasting impact. The experience gave me a glimpse of the true nature of our mind and body. It shaped my path forward in my personal and professional life in more ways than I can even fully grasp. And it gave me a firsthand experience of the mind-body connection, which is what I want to explore in this chapter. We have all heard of this connection, but studies are showing just how important it is to pay attention to it.

THE SCIENCE: OUR NERVOUS SYSTEM

According to Buddhist teachings, the secret of health for body and mind isn't to mourn for the past or worry about the future. It's to live in the present moment wisely and earnestly. Of course, this is easier said than done. Most of us spend a significant amount of our mental energy thinking about things that have already happened or are yet to happen, which leads to an inordinate amount of stress. In turn, that stress is a barrier to happiness.

We all want to be happy, but most of us don't know what that means. Psychologists and neuroscientists have studied the physiological, pharmacological, and behavioral aspects of happiness, identifying an area of the brain called the *nucleus accumbens* as our pleasure center. It secretes dopamine, the feel-good neurotransmitter. In other words, the secret to happiness lies somewhere in the brain. Besides the usual hedonistic pleasures that stimulate dopamine secretion, meditation has a similar effect on our brain circuitry. Studies have demonstrated that a meditation practice enhances brain volume in areas of the brain that are associated with happiness.[1]

If happiness isn't enough of an incentive, how about better physical health? A recent study at the Benson-Henry Institute for Mind Body Medicine at Massachusetts General Hospital found that people who meditated over an eight-week period had a striking change in the expression of 172 genes that regulate inflammation, circadian rhythms, glucose metabolism, and blood pressure.[2] No wonder meditation helps with a variety of conditions, especially the ones worsened by stress. These include anxiety, depression, pain, insomnia, post-traumatic stress disorder (PTSD), irritable bowel syndrome, fibromyalgia, food cravings, addictions, and more.[3]

To understand what stress does to your body, you need to understand the nervous system, which is made up of the brain and all the nerves that connect it to each organ and cell in the body. This network of nerve cells transmits information from the brain to the rest of the body, forming the basis of the mind-body connection. Since our liver, stomach, and kidneys don't have eyes or ears, they rely on our brain to tell them how to function. In fact, every cell in the body looks for its marching orders from the brain.

We're constantly assessing our environment through our senses, looking for any sign of danger. The brain decides whether the information gathered through sight, smell, taste, sound, and touch warrants attention. If it senses danger, it immediately sends a signal to the rest of the body. To accomplish this task efficiently, our nervous system has evolved with just two modes of operation. Even though the nerves, the organs, and the brain cells are the same, they act very differently, depending on which part of the nervous system is active.

The two modes of our nervous system are called the *sympathetic* system, which is the fight-or-flight mode, and the *parasympathetic* system, the rest-and-digest mode. Think of them as gears in a car. The car can either go forward or in reverse, depending on which gear it's in. Most of the time, we operate our car in drive and move forward; that's the default mode. Our nervous system's default mode is the rest-and-digest state. We cruise along through our daily life until we sense danger. Then we shift into fight-or-flight mode.

Every organ and every individual cell in our body behaves differently, depending on which mode we're in. For example, when we're run by our sympathetic system in fight-or-flight mode, our body acts as though we're running from a lion. Extra blood flows to our heart, lungs, and legs so that we can run as fast as possible. Our heart rate, blood pressure, and blood sugar shoot up, along with adrenaline and our major stress hormone, cortisol. At the same time, our sympathetic system turns off nonvital functions such as digestion and sex drive. While in that mode, all we care about is survival. This all makes sense if we think about our ancestors, who needed the fight-or-flight mode to survive starvation, bitter cold, severe weather, and predators.

The question is whether our stress is external or internal. External factors that cause stress on the body include extreme weather conditions, an infection, or a car accident. Fight-or-flight mode comes in handy as it tries to help us overcome life-threatening situations. All living creatures rely on this part of the nervous system to survive.

Survival, of course, is a good thing, so it might seem strange that this mode can also be a big problem.

WHAT GOES WRONG?

Let's say you're sitting in your bedroom, reading a book. Suddenly, the fire alarm goes off. Your senses send the information to your brain, which alerts every cell in your body that it's time to shift into fight-or-flight mode. A surge of adrenaline increases your heart rate and blood pressure, sending blood to your legs as it dilates your pupils to let in more light. This is followed by a release of cortisol. Again, all these responses happen to help you get out of dangerous situations.

If you experience a car accident, surgery, or illness, a few days of high cortisol helps you recover faster. Studies have shown that short-term stress boosts the immune system. Our mind and body can adapt to acute stress, which is what fight-or-flight mode has evolved to support.

But imagine that you have an *internal* fire alarm that goes off all the time. Your adrenaline lasts only for a few minutes, so as your brain senses danger, it triggers your adrenal glands to release cortisol to keep you in fight-or-flight mode—almost all the time.

Most of us may no longer have lions chasing after us, but our modern lifestyle is now the beast we fight daily. Our nervous system snaps into fight-or-flight mode the moment our alarm goes off in the morning, and we stay there while we're rushing to get to work, dealing with our difficult boss or clients, and picking up the kids after school. While these daily events don't pose imminent danger, our mind reacts to them as if they were a matter of life or death. These are what I call "internal" or self-created causes of stress. In this case, fight-or-flight mode becomes our default rather than the rest-and-digest mode that *should* be our default.

This chronic stress response leads to long-term elevation of cortisol. Then our mind-body connection goes haywire, as if we're pressing the panic button repeatedly. Higher levels of cortisol are associated with elevated mortality risk in older people, along with an increased risk of osteoporosis, high blood pressure, diabetes,[4] and heart disease.[5] Too much cortisol can also worsen anxiety, depression, digestive problems, headaches, insomnia, pain, weight gain, and memory issues.[6]

Research shows that the relationship between psychosocial stressors and disease is affected by a variety of factors. These include the nature, number, and persistence of the stressors, as well as our biological vulnerability (genetics and constitution), the resources we have available to help us, and our learned patterns of coping.[7]

This is why, during the first visit with a new patient, I prioritize learning about their stress level. It's one of the four pillars of integrative medicine: diet, exercise, sleep, and stress management. Stress is often the root cause of other problems. If it isn't addressed, we might not be able to follow a healthy diet, since high levels of stress hormones change our metabolism and even food cravings. We're also less motivated to exercise, and high stress hormone levels can prevent us from losing weight and increasing muscle tone. And we all know how stress can affect the quality and quantity of sleep.

Unfortunately, chronic stress has been on the increase in recent years. Since the COVID-19 pandemic and numerous other events in our country and the rest of the world, our lives have largely turned upside down. As if our usual levels of personal stress related to money, personal relationships, and health weren't enough, we now have existential threats like viruses, climate change, soaring inflation, and wars to worry about. The most recent Stress in America™ poll conducted by the American Psychological Association (APA) revealed that more than 80 percent of Americans report high levels of stress. "The number of people who say they're significantly stressed about these most recent events is stunning relative to what we've seen since we began the survey in 2007," says Arthur C. Evans, Jr., Ph.D., APA's chief executive officer.[8]

The effects of stress on our mind and body are certainly of great concern. On top of that, how we cope with chronic stress can further exacerbate the ill effects. For instance, the most recent APA survey confirmed that unhealthy coping behaviors under stress have become entrenched, and as a result, many people experience a continued decline of mental and physical health. Close to half of adults in the U.S. (47 percent) said they became less active than they wanted to be after the COVID-19 pandemic started, and close to three in five (58 percent) reported experiencing undesired weight changes. More than one in five Americans (23 percent) said they drank more alcohol.

If you want to enjoy optimal health, it's important to alleviate stress as much as possible. Let's explore two of the most common symptoms or conditions of chronic stress.

Common Symptom/Condition #1:
Anxiety and Depression

I think of the parasympathetic system as the yin energy of our nervous system and the sympathetic system as the yang energy. A balance between the two is ideal. We should be able to intentionally tap into either mode as needed. A problem arises when we unconsciously and repeatedly tap into flight-or-fight mode, which throws off the balance between yin and yang. Stress leads to too much yang energy.

When we're chronically stressed, the sympathetic nervous system may be continuously activated without the normal counteraction of the parasympathetic nervous system. Our immune system then responds with increased levels of pro-inflammatory proteins called *cytokines*. As these inflammatory cytokines accumulate, they have a neurotoxic effect on the brain, rendering it susceptible to depression.[9] The mechanism behind chronic stress and depression is very similar, as they can both be related to inflammation. It's no surprise that people with depression are often found to have high levels of inflammation.

No wonder many of my patients describe depression as something they feel in both their brain and their body. It's almost like having a low-grade flu every day; our body releases inflammatory cytokines when we're fighting a virus as well. Symptoms like chronic fatigue, body aches, and lack of motivation go hand in hand with depression. Therefore, when we address mental health, we need to pay more attention to the mind-body connection.

Anxiety is another mental health condition that's either caused by or exacerbated by chronic stress. In Ayurveda, anxiety relates to an imbalance in the vata dosha that often manifests as fearfulness and worry. In Chinese medicine, it's related to an imbalance in the kidney meridian. This isn't surprising, because the kidney meridian also includes our adrenal glands, which make the stress hormone cortisol. This is why chronic stress often depletes the kidney meridian, which, in turn, may manifest as anxiety.

According to Western medicine, the part of the brain called the *amygdala*, which is associated with fear and anxiety, is chronically activated when we're stressed. It's the primitive part of the brain that we have in common with other animals. Researchers have found that the local effects of chronic stress within the amygdala are likely to lead to an overactive circuit relating to fear and anxiety.

In other words, when we're stressed and act out of fear and anxiety, we're using the more primitive part of the brain, and this limits our ability to use the more advanced parts (the hippocampus and medial prefrontal cortex) involved in memory, fear inhibition, and cognitive thinking.[10] No wonder we make stupid mistakes when we're stressed and anxious. Whether you forget your keys or make a mistake at work, you can blame your amygdala the next time it happens.

Common Symptom/Condition #2: Stress Eating

When we're in fight-or-flight mode, our digestion is weak because we produce less saliva, enzymes, and stomach acid. Our gut either slows down, making us constipated, or it becomes overactive, sending us to the bathroom repeatedly. Our blood pressure, heart rate, and blood sugar remain high, setting the groundwork for developing high blood pressure, heart disease, and diabetes. High cortisol levels also cause us to crave more sugar and gain weight, especially belly fat, which is hard to shed.

The reason for this seemingly irrational behavior is that the amygdala cares only about survival. This animalistic part of the brain is motivated by fear and food. The food is to ensure we have enough calories to survive, and the fear is to make sure we avoid dangerous situations. If we want to train animals, we often use food or fear to motivate them. We can try reasoning with our dog that peeing in the house isn't a good idea, but treats are what will get the job done.

When we use the more primitive part of the brain, we know certain behaviors aren't good for us, but we do them anyway. We all know we should eat a salad rather than a candy bar, but when we're stressed, we bypass the more advanced parts of the brain for the primitive amygdala, succumbing to our cravings.

Research has shown that people tend to seek high-calorie, high-fat foods during periods of stress, and our bodies store more fat during stress than when we're relaxed.[11] That's a double whammy no one wants.

Despite our best intentions and knowledge, stress eating becomes our Achilles' heel. Even if you buy the healthiest food, chew it well, and eat at the right times, your diet can go south if you're stuck in fight-or-flight mode. Luckily, there are solutions to mitigate the impact of our stressful lives on the mind-body connection.

THE SOLUTION: OPTIMIZE THE MIND-BODY CONNECTION

Since we know that every cell in our body takes its marching orders from the brain, it makes sense that balancing the mind-body connection is an essential component of our well-being. In our modern lifestyle, our mind is in a constant state of turmoil, trying to juggle multiple tasks day and night. How can we thrive when we're simply trying to survive the stress?

When we're young, we're taught all sorts of subjects in school, from reading and writing to math and geography. Yet, we never learn how to cope with stress. It's inevitable in life, but we're supposed to figure out how to handle it on our own. Wouldn't it be amazing if we were trained at a young age how to recognize and deal with stress?

When I discuss stress-management techniques with my patients, they inevitably ask me about meditation. However, the Western concept of meditation is misleading. We immediately conjure a perfect image of someone sitting cross-legged on the floor in a quiet room with incense and sitar music. Living up to this image can be daunting.

The Eastern concept of meditation is quite simple. *Any activity during which you're fully present becomes meditation.* It isn't the activity that determines whether you're meditating; it's your attention that matters. You can be sitting in a dark room with the right music and an aromatherapy diffuser, but if your mind is going a hundred miles per hour while reviewing your to-do list or recounting the events of your day, you're not meditating. On the other hand, daily household chores like cooking or doing laundry can be meditative if done with intention and full awareness.

Few of us do this automatically—we can go through our whole day without being present for a single moment. It's like driving on a highway for hours, not realizing how you got from point A to point B. Wandering mentally into the past or future causes a lot of stress on our brain. It's the happiest when we're simply in the moment. Therefore, instead of going into a long discussion about meditation, I want to give you some simple tools for it. If you perform these techniques correctly with your full attention, you'll indeed be meditating.

Studies have shown that there are many ways we can destress and induce the relaxation response. For instance, deep breathing, guided imagery, and progressive muscle relaxation have all been found to be effective ways to promote psychological and physiological states of relaxation.[12] Let's look at each of these techniques, as well as a couple of others.

Use Guided Imagery

Do you ever go to your happy place when you feel overwhelmed? I love asking my patients what their happy place looks like. It's an overlooked coping mechanism when dealing with stress and anxiety. It might seem juvenile to escape to an imaginary land away from our problems, but it can genuinely help. Many studies support the use of guided imagery as an effective tool to help with symptoms of anxiety like tension headaches, abdominal pain, musculoskeletal pain, and postoperative recovery.[13]

Nature-based guided imagery exercises are especially effective in treating anxiety.[14] Those of us who live in urban settings often suffer from nature deficiency; being in nature is a powerful way to trigger the relaxation response. When you can't surround yourself with trees and birds, the least you can do is imagine them. If your mind thinks you're frolicking in a forest, the rest of your body will follow suit. Such is the wonder of the mind-body connection!

There are several excellent apps and websites with guided imagery exercises that you can use. Pick a setting you find most relaxing. Dedicate 15 to 20 minutes to it at any time during the day, and you will see how the stress begins to melt away.

Journal

Have you ever felt weighed down by your thoughts? Most of us carry too much information and troubling, deep-seated emotions in our heads. Journaling can help lighten the load a little, because it helps us clarify our thoughts and feelings and solve problems, and serves as a place of catharsis for painful emotions. According to Eastern medicine, our mind gets "sick" due to unprocessed thoughts and emotions. This leads to illness in the body. Studies have shown that journaling is even effective at improving cognitive function.[15]

It has also been found to reduce mental distress, anxiety, and depression while improving overall well-being,[16] and it can improve medical conditions such as asthma and arthritis.[17] Journaling has also helped my patients alleviate chronic pain, anxiety, and insomnia.

If you're new to journaling and don't know where to start, let me give you a few tips. Remember that your writing isn't meant to be a literary masterpiece; it's simply a place to park your thoughts and emotions. Don't get bogged down by your grammar or choice of words.

If writing about deep-rooted emotions or traumatic experiences is too painful, work with a therapist to find other topics. You can also start with easier topics to see how you feel.

If you tend to ruminate about events, such as things you said or didn't say, start by simply recounting the events of your day. Narrate what time you woke up, what you ate, and how you felt, and leave it at that.

If you have a hard time falling asleep because you're a busy bee with a long to-do list, journal about what you managed to get done. Too often, we focus on what we *didn't* accomplish. Once you feel comfortable accounting for what you complete, try adding your goals in your journal.

A gratitude journal is also a great place to start.[18] Studies have found that giving thanks and counting blessings can help us sleep better,[19] lower stress,[20] and improve our relationships.[21]

I find journaling to be a powerful tool for setting an intention. When the pen meets the paper, it adds substance to our intentions and helps us shape them. Then it becomes easier to visualize them.

Especially now that we spend so much time on our electronic devices, writing in a journal can be grounding and nostalgic. For those who find comfort in technology, however, there are plenty of ways to journal on a device.

Try Progressive Muscle Relaxation (PMR)

PMR is a relaxation technique that was developed by Dr. Edmund Jacobson in the 1920s. The idea behind it is that mental stress often manifests as physical tension. By sequentially tensing and relaxing different muscle groups, we encourage relaxation and strengthen the mind-body connection.

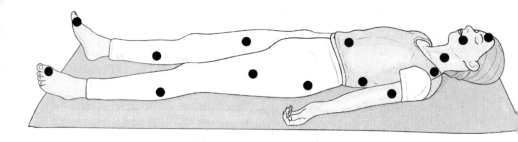

When you're more stressed, you're likely to hold tension in certain parts of your body such as your jaw, neck, and back. As you actively relax these muscle groups, you retrain your brain by sending different signals than the usual stress signals. It might feel odd at first, but over time, you'll notice a difference.

PMR is particularly helpful for insomnia. Often, I prescribe 20 minutes of this exercise to be done in bed in preparation for sleep. By actively triggering the relaxation response, our mind stops wandering and focuses inward. The brain is much more likely to quiet down and be present, which allows for an easier transition into deeper stages of sleep. No wonder the American Academy of Sleep Medicine rated it as an effective nonpharmacologic treatment for chronic insomnia.[22]

Many studies support PMR to alleviate anxiety as well.[23] It has been shown to be effective for treating tension headaches, migraines, temporomandibular joint disorder (TMJ), neck pain, backaches, high blood pressure, insomnia, and bipolar disorder.[24]

Here's a handy guide to get you get started with PMR.

1. Get comfortable: Make sure you're in a quiet and relaxing environment. Sit or lie down in a comfortable position.

2. Breathe deeply: Take a few deep breaths, inhaling through your nose and exhaling through your mouth.

3. Tense and relax your muscles: Starting with your toes, tense them and the muscles in your feet as

hard as you can. Hold the tension for a few seconds, and then release the tension. Feel the relaxation in your muscles.

4. Move up your body: Tense and relax each muscle group for a few seconds before moving on to the next one, going from your calves to your thighs, buttocks, stomach, back, arms, and hands.

5. Relax your shoulders and neck: Tense your shoulders by lifting them up to your ears, holding for a few seconds, and then releasing. Rotate your head slowly from side to side, feeling the tension release from your neck.

6. Focus on your breathing: Take a few deep breaths, inhaling through your nose and exhaling through your mouth. As you exhale, imagine the tension leaving your body.

7. End the exercise: Take a few more deep breaths and stretch your muscles gently. If you've been lying down, take your time getting up.

There are also several apps and videos available that can walk you through this 15- to 20-minute exercise. I highly recommend doing it at night as you get ready for bed.

Practice Mindful Eating

Addressing stress through mindful eating techniques can be our savior. In my practice, I teach patients to take a few deep breaths before they start a meal. This simple technique is powerful because it activates the vagus nerve, which can help us shift from fight-or-flight to rest-and-digest mode.

Eating mindfully has a vital impact on our cravings and sensation of feeling full. When we sit down in front of the TV with a bucket of popcorn or chips, we can go through a whole bag before realizing the damage we've done. If I asked you to sit in a quiet room without your phone or TV to distract you while eating a whole bag of popcorn or chips, you might have a hard time finishing that much. It's in eating mindlessly that we use the more primitive part of our brain and engage in behaviors that bring us instant gratification. If we do this time after time, it becomes our default mode of operation and changes our brain circuitry.[25]

Imagine participating in a hot-dog-eating contest. You're busy shoving hot dogs in your mouth, barely chewing them, and swallowing so quickly that your brain doesn't have a chance to figure out what's happening. Before it can catch up, you've already downed a dozen hot dogs.

Now imagine going to a Michelin-star restaurant for your birthday to splurge on a seven-course dinner. That may sound like a lot of food, but I've learned that the more Michelin stars a restaurant has, the smaller the portions are. When the first course arrives, it's no bigger than your thumb and costs more than a full dinner at Olive Garden. The waiter walks you through the story behind this morsel of food, which is a piece of gastronomic art on your plate. You can't wait to close your eyes, take a bite, and try to taste every ingredient. As the next few courses arrive, you're surprised you're already full, even though the total amount of food you ingested was less than one hot dog. What kind of culinary chicanery is this?

Your brain isn't playing tricks; it's simply responding to the signals it receives as you relish each bite. Unfortunately, our habit of "fast" food has extended to not just *what* we eat, but *how* we eat.

The moral of the story is that we should enjoy all our meals as if we're dining at an expensive Michelin-star restaurant. Wherever our mind goes, the body will follow, so it's important to chew our food well and take the time to notice its tastes, textures, and temperature. When we eat food mindfully, paying attention to its sight and smell, we activate the more evolved prefrontal cortex of our brain. This allows us to make better decisions about what we eat, how we eat, and how much we eat.

It takes about 20 minutes for our brain to realize we're full.[26] Slower, mindful eating helps regulate the amount of hormones such as ghrelin and leptin that send the brain signals of hunger and satiety respectively.[27] Then we receive the message that we're full before we mindlessly finish an entire bag of chips. Not only that, but we might also fight off weight gain and diabetes.

In a study published in the *British Medical Journal*, researchers asked almost 60,000 Japanese men and women with diabetes to categorize their eating speed. Not surprisingly, 37 percent categorized themselves as fast eaters, 56 percent as medium-paced eaters, and 7 percent as slow eaters. The major finding of this study was that changes in eating speed can affect the risk of obesity and diabetes. Those who ate at a slow speed were 42 percent less likely to be obese, and people who ate at a normal speed were 29 percent less likely to be obese.[28]

Food can be medicine or poison, depending on our mental state when we ingest it, which dictates how our body processes it. Eating while in a state of gratitude and mindfulness triggers a response in our body that significantly enhances our gut health.[29]

Jenny's Story

When Jenny came to me for weight loss, she expected me to place her on a strict diet and exercise regimen. During her initial consultation, I learned that she was very knowledgeable about nutrition and had already started cutting out processed foods, sugar, and red meat. She was also working out five days a week with a trainer, yet not seeing the results she wanted to. I was impressed with the changes she had already made, especially since she was a busy mom with two young kids and a full-time job.

I quickly realized, however, that Jenny was always on the go. She used to be a slow eater, but since having kids and working, she'd learned to finish her meals in a matter of minutes. Besides stress playing a role in her weight gain, I also suspected that the shift in the speed of eating was involved. She had no idea what or how many calories she was eating while on the go. She also had a habit of overeating at night, since it was the only time she could unwind. Instead of burdening her with restrictive diets or asking her to work out even more, I simply had her focus on mindful eating.

In place of a food journal, I asked Jenny to take a picture of all her meals. We focused on slowing down, chewing her food well, and paying attention to the tastes, textures, and aromas. I advised her to serve dinner on three different plates. This was tedious at first, but she quickly realized how much it helped her slow down the pace of eating. She spent more time chewing and ended up skipping the third plate because she registered as already full by the time she got to it.

Two months later, she reported hitting her weight-loss goal, even though she had reduced the number of days she was exercising to four instead of five days a week. Since she knew I would be reviewing the photos of her meals, she consciously stayed away from unhealthy foods and took Instagram-worthy pictures. She also spent a few more minutes dressing up her food, which automatically made her connect with what she was about to eat. Instead of dreading the decision about what to put on her plate, she began looking forward to it. It gave her a chance to channel her creativity and enthusiasm for how she nourished her body.

Adopt a Pet

There's a reason why dogs have been our best friends since eternity. Pets like dogs have a positive impact on our stress levels. This is why pet therapy is used in hospital settings to bring a smile to everyone's face. There's nothing more adorable than a golden retriever strolling the hallway of a hospital with a photo ID badge, reveling in all the attention. In one study, just a 10-minute visit by a therapy dog in the emergency room helped patients reduce their pain, anxiety, and depression while improving their well-being.[30] Other studies have revealed that even a brief interaction with a pet can significantly lower cortisol levels. According to the CDC, research shows that the bond between pets and their owners can lead to decreased blood pressure, cholesterol and triglyceride levels, feelings of loneliness, anxiety, and symptoms of PTSD. Pet ownership also offers more opportunities for exercise and outdoor activities, better cognitive function in older adults, and more chances to socialize.[31] If the health benefits of spending just a few minutes with pets could be squeezed into a pill, it would be a blockbuster drug.

Sixty-eight percent of American households have pets, so the key to reducing their stress and improving their health might be already living under their roof. Over the past 10 years, the National Institutes of Health has partnered with the Mars Corporation's Waltham Centre for Pet Nutrition to fund research studies on how pets can bring health benefits. It doesn't have to be a cat or dog. Other types of pets, such as fish and guinea pigs, can also be beneficial.[32]

Marwan Sabbagh, M.D., who has been a director of Cleveland Clinic's Lou Ruvo Center for Brain Health, said, "Simply petting an animal can decrease the level of the stress hormone cortisol and boost release of the neurotransmitter serotonin, resulting in lowered blood pressure and heart rate and, possibly, in elevated mood."[33] This just might be my favorite way of boosting the mind-body connection.

TIPS FOR REDUCING STRESS AND STRENGTHENING THE MIND-BODY CONNECTION

We just reviewed several different ways that can help you get out of fight-or-flight mode and into rest-and-digest mode. These techniques are a lot more effective than most people realize, not to mention safe. Often, we turn to medications or unhealthy ways of coping with stress. Instead, I strongly encourage you to add these techniques to your toolbox.

- Dedicate 10 minutes every night before bed to any of the above-mentioned practices. Here's a list of apps you can use to get started:
  - Calm
  - Headspace
  - Insight Timer
  - Ten Percent Happier Meditation

- • Buddhify
- • Simple Habit
- • Unplug

- Besides these apps, there are excellent free videos and audios online that you can use. I often refer patients to the Whole Health website by the U.S. Department of Veterans Affairs (www.va.gov/wholehealth/). It has wonderful free resources.

- The key is finding a practice that suits you and sticking to it. You'll be amazed what 10 minutes before bed can do to improve your sleep, mood, and overall health.

CHAPTER 8

THE BREATH
OF LIFE

After my medical residency, I spent countless hours studying Eastern medicine. I took courses, read books, and experimented with many techniques on myself and my husband, who played guinea pig for me. I had to learn a whole new side of medicine that I wasn't exposed to during my conventional clinical training. But books are never enough; I had to experience the knowledge through all my senses. So I decided to combine my love of travel with my love of medicine. Silent meditation retreats, trekking in the Amazonian jungle, and meeting Buddhist monks in some of the most remote parts of the Himalayan Mountains were far more exciting than sitting in a library. What I learned from these adventures dramatically transformed the way I see the human body and how I practice medicine.

One particular experience blew my mind. While in India a few years ago, I learned about an Ayurvedic practitioner who came from a long lineage of *vaidyas*, or Ayurvedic doctors. His approach is time-tested, with many successes. He even makes his own herbal medicines the same way they've been made for generations.

I figured the best way to learn in this scenario was to become a patient myself, so I made an appointment. Contrary to the process that my patients must go through, this was pretty straightforward. There were no long forms to fill out, no apps to download, and no barrage of text message reminders. This meant, however, that he didn't have much information about me besides my name and phone number.

I expected him to ask me questions about my health, check my tongue and pulse, give me a diagnosis, and recommend a treatment plan. Instead, we simply engaged in small talk for several minutes. After that, he paused for a moment and closed his eyes as if meditating. About a minute later, he opened his eyes and casually told me about my health from birth until that moment.

For a second, I thought I was in the wrong place. Perhaps I had come to a psychic or an astrologer instead of an Ayurvedic healer. As he went on about my health history, I tried to figure out where he had obtained the information. He just smiled as I expressed my astonishment. "I'm no magician; I'm simply present," he explained. By observing my body language, how I spoke, and, most important, how I breathed throughout our conversation, he had learned everything he needed to know. After that, to humor me, he examined my pulse and tongue. It was a true aha moment for me.

I learned from him that by simply observing someone's breath, I can find more information than any modern MRI or lab test can tell me. Most important, it can reveal not only what's going on in the body but also the mind and spirit. Our breath is what links our mind and body.

In fact, when I'm asked for my most important health advice, my answer is always the same: *breathe*. It sounds strange, since all of us have been performing this task without fail since the day we were born. But breathing is far more than an exchange of oxygen and carbon dioxide. Our breath, also known as *prana* or *qi*, is the vital energy that sustains all of us and harmonizes our body, mind, and spirit. For thousands of years, yogis and monks have known the power of the breath. The entire practice of yoga is based on first mastering the breath in order to master the body, which will eventually lead to mastering the mind. Monks and yogis spend decades in that pursuit.

According to yogic philosophy, there are eight steps to nirvana—the ultimate liberation from the cycle of birth and death. The first four steps focus on moral, ethical conduct and physical health. Once a strong foundation is created through these steps, we can focus on the later four steps toward spiritual advancement.[1] There are no shortcuts to this process.

Our mind and senses often interfere with peace. We've all experienced our monkey mind getting the best of us. It's the root cause of our stress and anxiety. If we want to achieve ultimate peace, we have to master the mind. Yoga is the science of life, laying down the path to ultimate peace through optimizing physical health by practicing physical postures called *asanas*. After that comes mastering the breath through the practice of breathing exercises called *pranayama*. Once the body is made strong and supple while the breath is controlled, the yogi can sit still and focus on the mind. Most of us try to jump ahead and immediately tackle the monkey mind. No wonder Westerners find it so hard to meditate.

Attaining nirvana might not be on everyone's bucket list, but peace certainly is. To get to that equanimous state, we must optimize our physical and mental health. Yoga gives us the tools we need, and they're accessible to all. If you can breathe, you can practice yoga. Don't be intimidated by social media yogis turning themselves upside down or into pretzels. Yoga is so much more than that.

There's also a lot more to it than speculation. The science bears out what yogis have known for centuries.

THE SCIENCE: THE VAGUS NERVE

Western medicine is recognizing the importance of breathing as a tool to optimize the mind-body connection. One of the ways to lower cortisol, get out of fight-or-flight mode, and connect the mind and body is to activate the vagus nerve, which runs from the brain through the neck and down into the abdomen. It's the king of nerves, as it controls the entire relaxation or parasympathetic response in our body. This means it also controls important functions such as our mood, immune system, digestion, heart rate, and sexual function.

As a result, researchers have been investigating vagus nerve stimulation as a treatment option for a variety of conditions, including depression, epilepsy, post-traumatic stress disorder, and inflammatory bowel disease. When we stimulate the vagus nerve, the level of cytokines that cause inflammation decreases and beneficial bacteria in the gut increase. This nerve acts like the messenger between the mind and the gut, as well as the rest of the body.

Yoga-based breathing exercises confer their health benefit by activating the vagus nerve, which explains why they improve symptoms like anxiety, depression, and stress while also optimizing gut health.[2] If you've ever been to a yoga or meditation class, you may have heard about the *chakras* in the body. These are energy centers, and when they're aligned and working optimally, the mind-body connection is balanced. When they aren't aligned, we're more vulnerable to diseases. If you look closely at the images that follow, you'll notice that the path of the vagus nerve aligns with the path of the chakras. In other words, when you activate

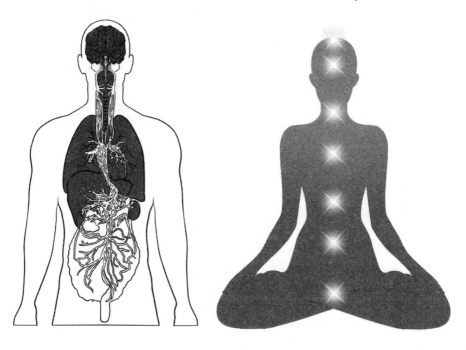

the heart chakra through certain yoga poses, it stimulates the vagus nerve at the level of the heart. This can help lower the heart rate and blood pressure. Western medicine's vagus nerve pathway is Eastern medicine's chakras; in the end, it's all the same.

We know we're on to something important when drug companies try to capitalize on knowledge that has been around for millennia. A simple breathing exercise can be a powerful tool in addressing symptoms like anxiety,[3] but there's no money to be made in teaching people how to breathe correctly. So why not make a product that stimulates the vagus nerve for you? All you have to do is place this small device underneath your collarbone and connect it to a wire that sends an electric signal to the vagus nerve in your neck. Such a device is currently FDA approved for epilepsy and the treatment of resistant depression. It's also being studied as a potential treatment for a myriad of conditions, such as migraines, fibromyalgia, rheumatoid arthritis, and even diabetes.[4]

Clearly our vagus nerve holds a tremendous amount of therapeutic potential. A small percentage of patients would benefit from such a stimulator, but for most people, simple breath training can lead to significant health benefits without any aggressive intervention. This is the best example of how Eastern and Western medicine can come together to optimize our well-being.

Let's explore in a bit more detail what goes wrong when we don't breathe properly and our vagus nerve isn't activated.

WHAT GOES WRONG?

Ever feel like your heart is beating out of your chest, your palms are sweaty, and your mind is racing? That's what a panic attack can feel like. If you've ever had one, you know it's a scary experience. For some people, it can be situational, while for others, the symptoms come out of nowhere. It's especially frightening when the trigger is unknown. The person feels like a sitting duck just waiting for the next episode to arise.

When we experience a panic attack, our mind-body connection has snapped into fight-or-flight mode with full intensity. The symptoms come from the adrenaline rushing through our veins.

But when the physical symptoms of fight-or-flight mode aren't as palpable, we might not be able to tell when our body is pumping out cortisol. When it's chronic, our body gets used to feeling stressed. Still, there are subtle physiological changes.

One of the main indicators is called *heart rate variability* (HRV). It's a measure of the variation in time between each heartbeat. This fluctuation is controlled by our autonomic nervous system. When we're stressed, the sympathetic nervous system causes HRV to go down. On the other hand, when we're relaxed, breathing well, and our vagus nerve is active, HRV increases.[5] Therefore, our goal is to train our nervous system to increase our HRV over time.

Bear in mind that HRV is different from our heart rate. We can take our pulse and see if our heart rate goes up when we're stressed or down when we're relaxed, but this measurement has several limitations. Everyone has a slightly different resting heart rate and cardiovascular conditioning. Many medications can also affect our heart rate, so it isn't an ideal measurement of stress response.

On the other hand, HRV is subtler and picks up even minor variations in our nervous system, so it's the measurement of choice for checking resilience and overall health. Studies have demonstrated positive changes in HRV from mindfulness, meditation, sleep, and especially physical activity.[6] Many wearable devices such as Fitbit and Apple Watch now give us real-time feedback about our HRV and, therefore, our stress level. For people who like objective data, there are a variety of ways to track HRV and see how diet, sleep, exercise, and overall lifestyle are affecting our health.

Besides serving as a cool feature in expensive wearable gadgets, HRV is also making waves in the medical research community. Whenever clinicians see a patient, we look for signs and symptoms that give us clues about risk factors for developing serious diseases. The sooner we identify these factors, the more time we have to intervene and hopefully delay or prevent the disease from occurring altogether. Prevention is always better than a cure.

The latest studies show that HRV can be used to predict outcomes and treatment response in a variety of conditions like depression,[7] PTSD,[8] kidney disease,[9] sepsis,[10] and heart disease.[11] It's even used to predict which patients with heart disease are at risk of sudden cardiac death—the leading cause of mortality in that patient population.[12] Think about HRV as a stress test for your nervous system. There's no need to run on a treadmill anymore to test your cardiovascular fitness level. We can simply hook you up to a simple device that tells us your HRV and predicts your risk for a host of conditions. There aren't many things in medicine that can give us so much data about your well-being and future risk, so this information is worth its weight in gold.

Let's look at two of the most common conditions related to the breath, the vagus nerve, and HRV: heart disease and post-traumatic stress disorder.

Common Symptom/Condition #1: Heart Disease

Our experience at the doctor's office hasn't changed much over the decades. We might have fancier machines to get the job done, but the information we obtain is essentially the same. Even though the latest research has demonstrated that the physiological measurement of HRV is a much better predictor of conditions such as heart disease, we have yet to put this into practice. We don't even need fancy equipment or special skills to check it. Somehow, in medicine, change is slow.

In my opinion, HRV is an important vital sign just like blood pressure or oxygen saturation. It can predict risk factors for so many conditions that it's worth checking—especially for heart disease, since it's the leading cause of death for both men and women of most racial and ethnic groups in the United States. About 659,000 people in the U.S. die from heart disease each year—that's one in every four deaths.[13] Shouldn't we be doing more to detect it sooner so that we can at least attempt to prevent it?

A study published in the journal *Circulation* looked at the predictive value of HRV for coronary heart disease and death in a large cohort of more than 14,000 patients. The researchers calculated HRV by checking a two-minute recording of each patient's electrocardiogram (EKG). They found that subjects with low HRV had an adverse cardiovascular risk profile and an elevated risk of coronary heart disease and death. The increased risk of death couldn't be attributed to a specific cause or explained by other risk factors.[14]

I wish we could give everyone an echocardiogram (a heart ultrasound) and stress test, but we just can't afford it. The dollar signs would add up quickly if we were to test millions of people in this way year after year, so a less invasive, cost-effective test like the EKG for HRV makes sense, especially when it also does a better job at showing risk.

A recent study evaluated more than a thousand patients who had low-to-intermediate pretest probability for coronary heart disease. These patients were lucky to get the whole workup to see if they had it. They underwent testing with a Holter cardiac monitor and either a stress echocardiography or a nuclear stress test. On top of the conventional testing, their HRV was also measured. Out of all the patients in the study, 6.3 percent were found to have signs of low blood supply to the heart (myocardial ischemia). This means that they were at a high risk of having a heart attack sooner or later. What was interesting was that after adjustment for heart disease risk factors and stress test results, low HRV was independently associated with a significant twofold increased likelihood for myocardial ischemia.[15]

Most of us know that chronic stress will affect our heart health in the long run, but the research shows exactly how this occurs. If we find ourselves in fight-or-flight mode too often with high cortisol coursing through our veins, our poor heart won't stand a chance. Stress does kill . . . and now we know how.

Common Symptom/Condition #2: PTSD

One statistic that haunts me, and should haunt every American, is that of the leading cause of death among our veterans: suicide. It's heartbreaking that the toll of trauma is sometimes as dangerous as the bullets and bombs they faced in combat.

PTSD is a complex neurobiological phenomenon character-ized by chronic dysregulation of reflexive survival behaviors. It leaves a lasting imprint on the mind, body, and spirit. The symp-toms can be grouped into three primary domains: (1) reminders of the exposure (including flashbacks, intrusive thoughts, and nightmares); (2) activation (including hyperarousal, insomnia, agitation, irritability, impulsivity, and anger); and (3) deactivation (including numbing, avoidance, withdrawal, confusion, dereal-ization, dissociation, and depression). Many of these symptoms are caused by an interplay within our hormone system, which includes cortisol and neurotransmitters such as serotonin and GABA (gamma-aminobutyric acid).[16]

Not too long ago, we believed that PTSD was simply a normal, if extreme, response to a traumatic situation. Now we know that how someone responds to a stressful situation is not only depen-dent on the stressor itself but also on the individual. Two people can experience the same traumatic event and have vastly differ-ent reactions to it.[17] So, it's important to identify risk factors to determine who is more likely to develop depression or PTSD after a traumatic event.

Again, HRV is a tool at our disposal. A recent study found that a lower HRV among veterans before they were deployed was asso-ciated with higher PTSD symptoms after their deployment.[18]

If we can do a better job of identifying people who are at higher risk of developing PTSD, we can intervene sooner. It isn't surprising that many mind-body intervention studies have been conducted with the veteran population. Mind-body practices like yoga breathing have been shown to reduce anxiety, depression, and anger while increasing pain tolerance, self-esteem, energy lev-els, the ability to relax, and the ability to cope with stressful situa-tions. These practices are also effective for a constellation of PTSD symptoms like intrusive memories, avoidance, and increased emo-tional arousal.[19]

Most of our current medications fail to address all these symptoms. Of course, it's also a challenge to make mental health services available to everyone who needs them most. Therefore, we need to increase awareness among clinicians and patients about these mind-body modalities and how they can be a valuable part of an effective treatment plan.

I personally had an experience of treating a man named Ed, who had PTSD. He was one of my first patients when I started my residency, and we developed a special bond over the years. His PTSD came from his time serving in the Vietnam War. Unfortunately, in those days, PTSD awareness and resources were severely lacking. As a result, many veterans turned to self-medicating with alcohol. Ed was no exception. He had tried to cut back on alcohol several times, and he suffered several health setbacks over the years.

I had come across several studies about PTSD treatment through vagus nerve stimulation and HRV monitoring, so I decided to see if these would benefit Ed. We did a biofeedback session, during which I connected him to a small heart rate variability monitor that displayed the results on my computer. During the session, we practiced guided imagery. I asked him to close his eyes and visualize a place or setting that he enjoyed, while I continued to monitor his results on the computer screen.

He did well, and his HRV went up as he felt calmer and more relaxed. Suddenly, however, his numbers went in the other direction and took several minutes to recover. At the end of the session, I asked him how he felt and if he had any negative thoughts during the guided imagery. He told me that he'd felt quite relaxed during the session, but he had a fleeting image of a warship when he tried to think of the ocean and beach. "I didn't pay much attention to it," he said.

Nevertheless, the microsecond reminder of that image put his nervous system into high alert. It was as if he were on the battlefield again at that moment, not in a doctor's office. He didn't have any overt symptoms of flashback or hyperarousal, but his HRV told me a more complex story. Even though he was able to brush away that image quickly, his nervous system took some time to quiet down. I was shocked to see how a very brief memory of the war could create dramatic fluctuations in his breathing pattern and heart rhythm, even though he didn't particularly *feel* stressed. We somehow get so used to snapping into fight-or-flight mode that we often don't pay attention to it.

THE SOLUTION: MANAGE STRESS WITH BREATHING AND BIOFEEDBACK

Ed's treatment focused on yoga-based breathing exercises and hypnotherapy. These modalities can help improve HRV by stimulating the vagus nerve and moving us out of fight-or-flight mode. Several studies have shown promising results with this approach in treating PTSD and even traumatic brain injury.[20]

As Ed found out, if we do nothing about our stress level, our cortisol will likely remain elevated, leading to a variety of chronic health conditions. Instead, if we intentionally train our nervous system, we can become resilient in the face of stressors.

It would be wonderful if we all learned to identify the signs and symptoms of stress at a young age. It would make us aware of the physiological and emotional changes that occur when we try to cope with challenges. Learning how to handle stress and building our resiliency could have a significant impact on all aspects of our lives.

According to the National Institutes of Health, *resilience* is "the ability . . . to bounce back from, or successfully adapt to stressors." This is true at the level of cells, organs, individual people, and societies. More research funding is being allocated so we can better understand the mechanisms underlying resilience and advance toward better prevention and treatment approaches.[21]

In my practice, teaching patients how to manage stress is a priority. Remember that stress management is one of the four main domains of integrative health, along with nutrition, sleep, and exercise. And it's the most important, because if we're stressed, it affects the other domains. In my opinion, learning how to manage stress is as important as learning how to walk.

Too often, we think of managing stress as a hobby and something to do in our leisure time. But it isn't enough to simply sit in a quiet corner with our eyes closed or download several apps with the best intention of using them daily.

My approach to stress management is intentional, methodical, and effective. I look at stress as I do any other disease. If I want to diagnose a condition, I must perform an assessment to figure out how bad it is, and I need objective and subjective data to make that determination. Let's say I suspect that one of my patients has high blood pressure. I'll observe their breathing and ask them whether they have symptoms like a headache, chest pain, or leg swelling. After that, I gather objective data by checking their blood pressure and HRV at several points in time. Once I have all the information, I make the diagnosis and come up with a treatment plan.

When it comes to stress, subjective interpretation can vary a lot from person to person, so we can never gauge the severity of the problem by subjective symptoms alone. Remember that fight-or-flight mode often becomes second nature to us when it's chronic for long enough. To encourage a patient to pay more attention to it, I must show them the proof. I mentioned that I performed a biofeedback session with Ed to obtain a better understanding of his nervous system. Let's talk more about what the term *biofeedback* really means and how anyone can use it to acquire an objective assessment of their stress level.

Self-Regulate with Biofeedback

To have a better understanding of how someone's nervous system is operating, we need to know how much time they're spending in fight-or-flight versus relaxation mode. When we're stressed, several physiological parameters change, such as our HRV, breathing rate, blood pressure, skin temperature, and sweat gland activity.[22] With the use of specialized equipment, we can gather data about our nervous system by measuring these subtle changes. Until recently, we believed that we had no control over these changes. However, research shows that isn't the case.

For example, when I traveled through remote parts of the Himalayas in Northern India, I encountered several Tibetan monks with extraordinary abilities. The temperature in this remote area can be so low that the cold makes it almost uninhabitable. Through meditation and breathing exercises, however, the monks there were able to raise or lower their body temperature at will. Researchers at Harvard have conducted experiments where cold sheets were placed on the monks, who sat in a room that was only 40 degrees Fahrenheit. The monks were somehow able to generate enough body heat to dry the ice-cold sheets within an hour.[23]

While the biofeedback we use may not be quite that dramatic, it's an effective self-regulation technique through which patients learn to voluntarily control what we once thought were involuntary body processes. Just like the monks, we can learn to control our breathing, heart rate, and body temperature. Think of biofeedback training as physical therapy for our nervous system. If we have knee pain after an injury, we see a physical therapist. If our nervous system is constantly on high alert due to stress, we should see a biofeedback therapist. They undergo specialized training to help patients get a glimpse of their nervous system, and they direct patients to use biofeedback to learn how to regulate their physiology in a healthy direction.

Even if you've never heard of biofeedback, I'll bet you've seen it in action on your TV screen. A lie detector test is a biofeedback device since it uses respiratory rate, sweat gland activity, and heart activity to determine if someone is stressed due to lying. Based on all the spy movies I've watched, I've learned that we can be trained to fool a lie detector test. This is the same idea behind what I'm doing with my patients. Of course, when we can control some of these body processes for the betterment of our health, it's a good thing.

Depending on your health goals, a biofeedback therapist might measure a variety of parameters, including the following:[24]

- *Brain waves:* This type of biofeedback therapy is also known as *neurofeedback.* Scalp sensors monitor brain waves, and expertise is required to interpret the data. Some of the newer devices on the market, such as the Muse headset, are making this technology more user-friendly.

- *Breathing rate:* This is monitored via a chest or abdominal strap. You might have seen these on athletes when they're training on a treadmill.

- *Sweat gland activity:* Sensors are attached around the fingers or wrist to measure the activity of the sweat glands and the amount of perspiration on the skin. This is often used in lie detector tests.

- *Temperature:* Sensors are attached to the fingers or feet to measure blood flow to the skin. When we're stressed or anxious, blood moves away from our extremities, toward the core of the body. This causes the temperature in our fingers and feet to go down. Mood rings change color in response to body temperature.

- *Muscle contraction:* Needle-like sensors go into our skeletal muscles like an IV to measure the electrical activity that causes muscle contraction. This can be cumbersome, so it isn't commonly used.

- *Heart rate variability:* This is the one I like to use. It's usually measured with a sensor on a finger or ear, but it can also be measured using a chest strap.

I wish everyone had access to biofeedback training, but the reality is that it's still a limited resource. Fortunately, new user-friendly gadgets are making biofeedback more accessible and affordable. One device that I use in my practice is a heart rate variability monitor called Inner Balance. It's easy to use with an app for most smartphones and tablets. The device itself is small and clips onto the earlobe, where it monitors heart rhythm and sends the data to the app for analysis. The app then interprets the beat-to-beat variation in our heart rhythm to provide a score that tells us about the activity of our vagus nerve. The more active our vagus nerve, the higher our HRV score is. The higher our HRV score, the less stressed we are.

Since the device captures data in real time, we can also see how our thoughts have a direct impact on our heart rhythm. My patients are amazed when they see how thinking about a work deadline instantaneously causes their score to dip, while thinking about their pet or child makes it go up. This data is so powerful because it's often the first time we see the mind-body connection in action. We can directly observe how one thought is powerful enough to change the way our heart beats, how we breathe, and even how our sweat glands operate.

Retraining your nervous system is serious business, however. I often compare it to training for a marathon. When you train for a grueling 26-mile run, you don't start by running 26 miles. You start with just a couple of miles every day. As you build your stamina, you're able to run longer distances over time. Imagine if I asked you to run in circles every day without tracking your time or distance. You wouldn't know if you were improving. To keep track of your progress, you need subjective and objective data. If I'm training for a race, I like to know the distance I'm running, my speed, and my heart rate.

Just like a runner, we need objective data about our stress level to tell us how we're doing, so that we can continue to make progress in the right direction. I find heart rate variability to be the most user-friendly and accurate of these tools, so I use it routinely to train patients to manage their stress and build resilience.

Biofeedback devices are similar to blood pressure devices. If our HRV is abnormal, we can use that information to try treatments that might improve it. Using a machine that tells us we're stressed is only the first step.

I often set concrete goals with my patients. If they're using the HRV monitor, we develop a personalized regimen and target scores week after week.

Now let's explore how the ancient wisdom of yoga-based breathing exercises can help us reduce stress, build resilience, and strengthen the mind-body connection through our breath.

Perform Breathing Exercises

If there's one skill I can teach someone to optimize their health, it's how to breathe correctly. Even though we're born with the ability to breathe, there's a lot of room for improvement. We take it for granted, but when done properly, the act of taking in oxygen and breathing out carbon dioxide helps us not only survive but also thrive. Just as the Ayurvedic doctor was able to tell me so much about my health by simply observing my breathing, you can learn a lot about your own body by simply watching how you breathe.

We hardly pay attention to our breathing, unless we're climbing up a few flights of stairs with someone else. We've all been there, trying to play it cool and pretend we aren't out of breath. In those moments, we become acutely aware of our breathing and the pumping of our heart. At any given time, if you paid close attention, you might notice how your thoughts, emotions, and activities constantly shape your breathing.

Since your breath is the link between your mind and body, you can use it to your advantage. But you may not realize that besides a mind-body connection, there's also a body-mind connection. Just as your brain can send signals to every cell in your body, your cells can also relay messages to your brain and influence its function.

Let's say you're walking down the street and see a nail on the ground. Your brain sends a signal to your legs to change your course and avoid stepping on the nail. If you aren't paying attention and never see the nail, your brain is oblivious to its presence. Then you step on it. Your brain knows you stepped on the nail because your cells and the nerves in your feet sent a signal to your brain.

This constant communication between the mind and body is mediated by the breath. The minute you step on the nail, you huff and puff in agony. That's a signal to the brain and the rest of your body that announces danger. In that moment, if you were able to consciously regulate your breathing (which would be easier said than done), you might feel less pain and discomfort. By changing your breath, you could dampen the danger signal to your brain, and more specifically to the areas of your brain that control the pain response. No wonder we're often told to take deep breaths when we're in pain.

Besides pain, our emotions have particular breathing patterns. Emotions aren't just psychological; they're also physiological. They occur because of activation of the muscular, cardiovascular, endocrine, and autonomic nervous systems.[25] Researchers have found that our respiratory patterns are not only influenced by emotions, but they also influence emotions in a bidirectional relationship between the body and mind.[26] Hence, breath training can be used to optimize the mind-body connection, as well as emotional regulation.

Sometimes our emotions get the best of us. We frequently react to situations based on habit instead of responding to them with intention. My patients often comment that after practicing breathing exercises, they notice a better ability to regulate their thoughts and emotions. As soon as they perceive irregularity in their breath, they bring it under conscious control. This allows them to be more present and respond to any situation, especially a stressful one, rather than overreact.

Let's take a moment to pay closer attention to your breath. Place one hand on your chest and one hand under your belly button. Close your eyes for a couple of minutes, and simply feel the movement in your chest and belly as oxygen comes in and carbon dioxide goes out through your nostrils. You'll probably notice that most of the movement occurs in your chest. We often breathe in this shallow way, sending air mostly to the upper part of our lungs. Yet, due to gravity, most of the blood is in the lower part of our lungs, so it makes more sense to send our air to that area. We want the oxygen to go where most of the blood is located. This will oxygenate the blood better and help get rid of more carbon dioxide.

Now try taking slow, deep breaths. You can tell if they're deep enough and oxygenating the lower part of your lungs, because when you breathe properly, you use your diaphragm, which is the most important breathing muscle. (It's a dome-shaped muscle that sits between your lungs and belly.) Then the lower lungs expand, pushing the diaphragm down and flattening it as the belly expands out.

Besides improving oxygen delivery to every cell in your body, this type of diaphragmatic breathing has another important advantage. The vagus nerve, which controls our relaxation response and helps us get out of fight-or-flight mode, passes right through the diaphragm. Therefore, every time you engage this breathing muscle, its movement massages and stimulates the vagus nerve.

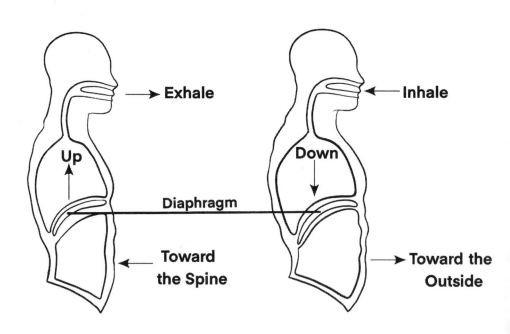

In yoga, pranayama comprises several breathing exercises. Each has various health benefits, as they all improve oxygenation in the body and strengthen the vagus nerve. Studies have shown that pranayama practice can have a positive effect on anxiety and brain function.[27] These findings were evident from functional MRI imaging after just four weeks of breathing practice.

You don't need to spend years practicing yoga, meditation, or breathing exercises. These simple techniques can have an instantaneous and long-lasting effect. All you have to do is get started and stick to the practice. Follow the tips below to improve your breathing. Whether we're looking for nirvana or simply optimal health, our journey begins and ends with the breath of life.

TIPS FOR BETTER BREATHING

These easy steps will not only improve your breathing, but they will also stimulate your vagus nerve, strengthen your mind-body connection, and help you move into rest-and-relaxation mode.

- Check in with your breath every hour. It simply takes a few seconds of your time. By paying closer attention to it, you'll have several opportunities to reset your mind-body connection. Instead of superficial breaths, diaphragmatic breathing will gradually become second nature to you.

- Try combining diaphragmatic breathing with guided imagery or progressive muscle relaxation exercises at night.

- For those of you who are inspired by the Tibetan monks, consider finding a yoga teacher who can teach you pranayama-based breathing exercises.

- For day-to-day application, I often encourage my patients to take three reset breaths every hour. You can do this when you're driving, in an elevator, or during commercial breaks while watching television. Simply take three deep breaths that expand your belly and oxygenate your lungs.

- Practice reset breaths whenever you're in a stressful situation. Whether you're about to take an exam, give a presentation, or in an argument with your loved one, simply breathe. Allow your vagus nerve to become activated, let your HRV increase, and enable the more advanced part of your brain to dictate how to respond instead of reacting on automatic.

- If you like, you can find a biofeedback specialist and/ or purchase an HRV sensor of your own.

PART III

• • • • • • •

SUSTAINING INTENTIONAL HEALTH

CHAPTER 9

THE 28-DAY RESET

No diet or workout plan can promise health and vitality. Our body is way too intelligent and already has the software it needs to bring us into balance. In that respect, I see it as much like my computer or cell phone. When they malfunction, my first course of action is to hit the Restart button. It allows the hardware and software to sync up again, often fixing at least half of the problem. If a few minutes and some patience can improve half of our technology woes, that's a pretty good return on our time investment.

Restarting a device won't fix significant issues like viruses, outdated operating systems, or hardware damage, but most of the problems we encounter aren't that serious. If we act at the earliest sign of any irregularity and perform maintenance and cleanup from time to time, we just might avoid the more serious problems.

Similar logic applies to the body. Just like you don't have to be a technology expert to fix common issues in the devices you use every day, you don't have to be a health expert to bring your body back into balance. Since you live with your body every day, you can detect minor issues before they're apparent to any health expert.

Think of this 28-day reset like restarting your computer. Regardless of why you need a reset—whether due to a chronic illness or mainly to increase vitality—it's a first step that's applicable to all. For almost every new patient I see, regardless of the reason for their consultation, this is the regimen I recommend. It's my way of syncing their hardware and software before I do anything else. After that, their body will have unlocked its inner intelligence so that any further diet or lifestyle changes I recommend will be far more effective.

The central concept behind this regimen is as simple as turning the computer off and on, but in our case, we need about 28 days to reset. But why do we need a reset in the first place?

BALANCE, NOT PERFECTION

Life happens, and nothing in our life is static, so it's natural that we need to reset from time to time. Think back to the last time you went on a weekend bender with friends or ate your way through the buffet on vacation. Or the time you went through a breakup or had a rough week at work and tried to drown your sorrows in a tub of ice cream or a bottle of wine. I don't have to tell you that these behaviors aren't the best for your health. What are you supposed to do? Stop living? Certainly not.

We often consider these life events as setbacks on our journey to optimal health. That's because we think perfection is the only choice. Somehow, we're all supposed to have a thin waistline and age gracefully like Paul Newman or Cher. Instagram models might have the luxury of making a living out of working out and drinking perfect protein smoothies, but that isn't the reality for most of us.

These idealized clips of wellness do less to inspire us and more often make us feel guilty. If we don't manage to work out or eat pristine meals every day, we feel guilty. If we indulge or stress eat, we feel guilty. This guilt slowly chips away at our self-esteem and determination. Comparison is indeed the thief of joy.

When it comes to health, trying to attain perfection is one of the biggest illusions, and we seem to be constantly bombarded with the idea. My aim in helping you learn more about your health is not to make you think you have to be perfect.

No one is perfect, and no one has to be.

My patients assume I have a picture-perfect diet, exercise every day, and never look at desserts. Nothing could be further from the truth.

I travel to Italy every year to eat my weight in pasta and drink more wine than water. And when I visit India, I enjoy the irresistible street food, even if I risk spending the next few days on the toilet. I live to eat, and I love to travel. I wouldn't give up either, even if I could live a decade longer. I stick to moderation most of the time, but hey, when in Rome. . . .

You might be wondering how I indulge and even overindulge occasionally while staying healthy. *It's all about balance.*

In Chinese medicine, health is a state of balance between the yin and the yang. It's never about perfection. When life gives you too much yang, bring in more yin, and vice versa. In other words, after a week of eating my way through Italy, I spend the following two weeks detoxing and eating a simple diet. I wish I could eat pasta forever, but if fasting after feasting can help me enjoy life's pleasures while keeping my body healthy, it's worth it!

With balance in mind, let's get to the nuts and bolts of your 28-day reset.

AN AYURVEDIC DETOXIFICATION RITUAL

If your body can reset and realign, it will work more efficiently to get rid of the toxins built up over the years. Once they're removed, you can start with a clean slate and nourish your body with nutrient-rich food, along with herbs to help it rebuild and rejuvenate.

We'll start by putting all the knowledge you've gained so far into practical, actionable steps. Each ancient secret you've learned is a rock upon which you'll build the foundation of health and vitality.

This regimen will also help you learn to pay close attention to your body so that you can identify imbalances before a doctor can detect them through a lab test or a CT scan. In order to feel youthful and blissful, and defy age and diseases, you must fix issues at the earliest sign of wear and tear before they become a bigger problem. This reset will help you achieve that goal. I developed it based on my personal experience and the knowledge I've gained in treating thousands of patients. Its foundation lies in the ancient process of panchakarma, the Ayurvedic detoxification ritual I described earlier.

Why choose this regimen over all the other programs that are available? There's no shortage of promises made by books and health experts to help you turn your life around in two weeks or two months. But this plan isn't about dieting. I won't promise eternal youth or a specific waist size. It's simply a Reset button to help you feel balanced and vital again.

Some of you reading this might feel like you're doing well. You don't suffer from any symptoms or diseases, so you may feel that you don't need to press Reset. But remember: It's always harder to fix things once they're broken. This regimen will help you maintain your good health. On the other hand, if you suffer from chronic fatigue, brain fog, gastrointestinal issues, inflammation in the body, hormone imbalance, or other chronic diseases that affect your quality of life, you can jump-start your health journey now.

Optimal Timing

According to Ayurveda, the best time to do any cleansing or detox ritual is in the fall or spring. All living organisms experience a significant shift in their metabolism during these times. This phenomenon is etched into our genes. It's how birds know to fly south in the winter and trees know to shed their leaves in the fall.

With our thermostats set at 70 degrees, we might not perceive the changes in seasons as much as our ancestors did. Yet, whether we realize it or not, even in the 21st century, our bodies naturally try to detox and prepare for new seasons. This transition can be much smoother if we facilitate the process by simplifying our diet and lifestyle. Not slowing down during this natural transition often affects our immunity and makes us more susceptible to allergies and cold viruses around those times of the year.

Modern science overwhelmingly supports this. A large study conducted at Cambridge University looked at the genes from more than 16,000 people from Northern and Southern Hemisphere countries such as the U.S., the U.K., Iceland, Australia, and the Gambia. The study collected blood and fat tissue samples and analyzed them in detail to look for seasonal variation in gene activity. Researchers found that more than a quarter of the 20,000-plus genes tested had different activity levels depending on the time of year. Some were more active in the winter versus the summer. This change affected blood cells, immune cells, and even fat cells.[1]

These findings aren't surprising, because we notice a seasonal change in many inflammatory conditions and even heart disease, which is aggravated in the winter. They also found that, depending on the season, the immune system changes its threshold for activation. For instance, in Europe, immune system genes are more active in the winter since viral illnesses are more common during that time of the year. Similar changes were noted in the Gambia during the rainy season, when mosquito-borne diseases are more common.

This research simply affirms what people practicing the ancient medical systems knew for thousands of years. They intuitively created a detox routine around certain times to help the body acclimatize better. This allowed their immune system and metabolism to transition into the next season, and by adapting to the body's changing needs, they could keep it in balance and maintain their vitality for years to come.

For menstruating women, I suggest starting the 28-day reset right after your period. Your body naturally slows down during your period, and your energy level tends to be low, so it isn't an ideal time for a detox.

Of course, avoid detoxification while you're pregnant or breast-feeding. Some of the herbs aren't good for you during this time, and you need to absorb the maximum amount of nutrients for you and your baby. For patients who are thinking of getting pregnant soon, I advise them to undergo the reset at least six months prior to trying to conceive.

Since life happens, you might need to use this reset regimen from time to time. Even though we clean our house regularly, we need a deeper clean periodically. This plan can be your go-to for keeping your body in better balance long term. I recommend it annually or semiannually, but you can use it any time you want to breathe vitality back into your body. Generally speaking, start the reset when you feel well, not during an acute illness or while you're recovering from an illness.

In any event, always consult with your physician before making any significant changes to your diet or lifestyle, even for a short time.

Ground Rules

Whenever I recommend this regimen to my patients, I'm obligated to remind them it isn't easy. If it were, it wouldn't work as well. It requires a discipline level that most of us aren't accustomed to. So let me prepare you for what's to come.

- Embark on this journey when you can commit your time and attention to it. Anything less than 100 percent isn't good enough for you.

- Remember the power of positivity when setting your intention. You'll see this in action over the next 28 days. You can set a specific intention for your reset, which will be your body's marching orders. Be very clear with yourself about what you want to accomplish. It isn't about "losing 50 pounds." Remember to focus on what you can control. Instead, you might intend to "give 100 percent attention to my body to help it heal" or to "be kind to myself."

- Be realistic with what you can do and what you can expect in return. The amount of effort, discipline, and focus you bring to the table is what you will get back. Instead of focusing on the outcome, however, choose to focus on your actions.

- Detoxification is like giving your body a decluttering makeover, but it's an emotional, as well as physical, process. You'll open boxes and closets that you haven't opened in a long time, and they might bring joy or sadness. At times, deep-seated emotions will surface, which can be triggering.

- Patience is indeed a virtue during the 28 days. Some of the diet and lifestyle changes will be new to you and will take some time to get used to. Be extra kind and supportive of yourself. When temptation gets in the way, remind yourself why you're doing it, and return to your intention.

- The process itself is the biggest reward. It will teach you more about yourself in less than a month than most of us learn in years.

THE RESET

The 28-day reset has four phases:

Preparation ▸ Detoxification ▸ Reintroduction ▸ Rejuvenation

Phase 1—Preparation: This is the initial step, which lasts a week. In my opinion, this is the most crucial step. The more you allow yourself to slow down and make your health your singular focus over the next 28 days, the better your results.

Phase 2—Detoxification: During this week-long step, you will further simplify your diet and lifestyle. Doing so will allow your body to shift gears. Instead of spending a lot of energy to break down food, your body can now focus on removing toxins that are a product of improper digestion—the root cause of all diseases. With a mono-diet, prolonged intermittent fasting, and detoxifying herbs, you can further enhance the cleansing process.

Phase 3—Reintroduction: You will slowly get back into your daily routine after the detoxification phase. Your body worked hard during detoxification, so it's important to reintroduce foods and increase your activity level gently. Doing it too quickly can overwhelm your body.

Phase 4—Rejuvenation: Once the toxins have been mobilized and eliminated, you're presented with a clean slate. You have the opportunity to consciously decide what you want to put back in your body. The addition of herbs and supplements will enhance the rejuvenation process because they'll be far more effective post-detox. This phase starts after 21 days and continues for months.

After completing the vitality regimen, you'll seamlessly transition into your 20-minute daily self-care routine, which you'll read about in the next chapter. Why stop at 28 days when you can continue to reap the benefits of this program for years to come? The daily self-care routine will help you continue the detoxification and rejuvenation process without the intense discipline of the reset.

Now that you have the lay of the land, let's explore the details of each phase.

Phase 1: Preparation

Abraham Lincoln once said, "Give me six hours to chop down a tree, and I will spend the first four sharpening the ax." Preparation is often the key to success, and that definitely holds true for the 28-day reset. The first step in jump-starting your health journey is to actually do *less*. It might be counterintuitive to our Western mindset, which is constantly programmed to do more, faster and better. But in this case, the less you do, the better results you'll yield.

In Eastern philosophy, doing less, simplifying the diet, becoming more mindful, and paying closer attention to the state of your body are of great importance. This philosophy allows you to prioritize the elimination of toxins before repair and regeneration. It's similar to buying an old house that's a fixer-upper. First you make sure it has a strong foundation. Then you fix the plumbing and electrical system, followed by painting and sprucing up with new furniture. If you jump ahead to paint the walls first, you have a house that's still going to fall apart.

Too often, people try to do it all at once. They change their diet dramatically and start taking bags full of supplements, hoping to reverse the damage done over the years. This 180-degree shift asks their body to work doubly hard to process too many supplements while also processing nutrients and toxins.

Instead, during the reset, your body can finally focus on healing, releasing toxins, and reducing inflammation while it stops playing *Whac-A-Mole* with unpredictable mealtimes, bedtimes, and stress levels. By simplifying your diet and lifestyle during this time, you support the natural processes ingrained in your DNA to help you repair and rejuvenate. Your job is to get out of your body's way.

Let's look at the diet I propose for this first seven days of the reset.

Diet

When it comes to dietary changes, the first rule is "do no harm." The primary rationale behind avoiding the foods in the first column is to give your digestive system a break. Foods such as wheat, dairy, and animal products use up most of your digestive fire. The harder a food is to digest and process, the more it's likely to trigger inflammation. Ingredients like high-fructose corn syrup and hydrogenated fats significantly overwhelm the body's detox machinery and cause inflammation. A simple rule of thumb is to eat foods that don't come in a box or contain more than one ingredient. This ingredient should be something our ancestors would have recognized. During the 28 days, it's important to be even more vigilant than usual.

	Foods to avoid	Reasons	Eat this instead
Gluten	Wheat, barley, rye, couscous, spelt, farro, kamut	• Hard to digest • Gluten sensitivity and intolerance are common	Gluten-free grains such as oats, rice, quinoa, millet, buckwheat, amaranth
Dairy	Milk, yogurt, cheese, butter Exception: ghee	• Hard to digest • Often contains hormones	Almond milk, oat milk, coconut milk, coconut yogurt, ghee
Animal products	Meat, seafood	• Takes too long to digest and process • Affects the gut microbiome • Contains hormones and antibiotics	Lentils, beans, tofu, edamame, honey
Processed foods	Potato chips, candy, soda, packaged desserts	• No nutritional value • Increases inflammation and insulin levels • Contains preservatives and artificial coloring	Fruits (fresh or dried), small number of nuts or nut butters
Alcohol, Caffeine, Drugs	Beer, wine, hard liquor, coffee, illicit drugs, marijuana	• Alcohol and drugs affect the liver, which is your main detox organ • Caffeine affects your adrenal glands	Non-caffeinated herbal teas, ginger, mint, jasmine, chamomile, CCF tea

There's ample research behind how eating a whole-food, plant-based diet is good for our overall health. It promotes the growth of good bacteria in the colon, reduces inflammation, and can even prevent colon cancer.[2]

Mindful Eating

The act of eating is far more than simply ingesting food. During the entire 28-day reset, pay even closer attention than usual to how and when you eat.

- Consume two to three meals per day, separated by at least three hours. Avoid snacking.

- Be mindful of your portion sizes. After a meal, your stomach should contain one-third solid food and one-third liquid. The other one-third should be left empty. A soup bowl holds around 10 ounces of liquid. Your stomach size is three times that. Hence, it makes sense to eat about two soup bowls' worth of food and leave another bowl's worth of space for the gastric juices to do their magic.

- Make lunch your biggest meal, with a lighter dinner that you eat earlier than usual.

- Drink plenty of warm water throughout the day, mostly between meals.

- To help stimulate digestion, drink one cup of ginger tea with meals and one cup of cumin, coriander, and fennel tea (CCF tea) after meals.

- Slow down, chew your food well, and avoid looking at screens while you eat.

Lifestyle

During the entire 28 days, continue your daily activities, such as work or school and household chores. But put anything outside of these necessities on hold as much as possible. This is not the time to start a new project, run a marathon, travel, or socialize too much. Instead, use this opportunity to look inward and learn more about yourself.

Think of it as an opportunity to recharge your battery. Remember that your senses are the biggest drain on your energy, so give them a break for these weeks. Keep time on social media and in front of the television to a minimum, because these activities are much more exhausting than we realize. Conserve your physical, mental, and emotional energy, along with those hours of your time.

Instead, read uplifting books, listen to soothing music, and write in your journal. These are great ways to supercharge your battery. If you have a meditation practice, dedicate more time to it than you normally would. Even if you've never meditated before, engage in deep breathing, long walks, or time in nature.

Continue regular exercise but avoid long, strenuous workouts. Instead, try more mindful movements like yoga, Pilates, or tai chi. Conserve your energy while improving circulation and flexibility with these gentle practices. The ideal time for exercise is in the morning. You can take a walk or engage in a gentle yoga nidra practice in the evening, which enhances relaxation and improves sleep.

Adequate sleep should be one of your top priorities. As you already learned, most of the metabolic activity pertaining to detox, repair, and rejuvenation occurs while we sleep. Try your best to get at least eight hours of restful, uninterrupted sleep.

Daily Routine

During the entire reset, strive to realign your circadian rhythm. We've already discussed how synchronizing our biological clock with the natural cycles can prevent heart disease,[3] mood disorders,[4] and even Alzheimer's disease.[5] Early to bed and early to rise will be your mantra for the duration of this regimen.

If your body knows what to do every day, it can do it efficiently. The preparation phase is all about laying this strong foundation in the form of a daily routine. I've provided an ideal schedule, which you can use as a blueprint to create your own.

Oral Care

Ayurveda places significant emphasis on oral care, which is believed to be intimately connected to our gut health. This isn't surprising, since our oral cavity houses the second largest microbiome after our gut. Any imbalance in the oral microbiome will perturb the gut as well. In fact, imbalances in the oral microbiome have been linked with rheumatoid arthritis, pancreatic cancer, diabetes, and heart disease.[6] We aren't far from the day when

Sample Daily Routine

6:00–6:30 A.M.	Rise Start your day by expressing gratitude and setting an intention for the day Oral Care: • Oil pulling with 1/2 teaspoon of coconut or sesame oil • Brush your teeth and floss like your dentist is watching • Tongue scraping (See the upcoming section for information about oil pulling and tongue scraping.) Drink 16 ounces of warm water; add lemon if you like A bowel movement should follow soon after
6:30–7:30 A.M.	Meditation Breathing exercises, as discussed in Chapter 8 Gentle workout of your choice: walking, biking, yoga, Pilates, or tai chi Shower
8–9 A.M.	Breakfast Ideas: • Fresh fruits or fresh-pressed juice with ginger • Steel-cut oatmeal with coconut sugar, cinnamon, raisins, and/or almond butter • Congee
12–1 P.M.	Lunch Ideas: • Vegetarian chili and quinoa • Chickpea flour pancake with mushroom filling • Coconut curry with cauliflower rice • Falafel wrap with butternut squash soup • Veggie burger and roasted sweet potato fries • Cup of ginger tea with your meals to stimulate digestion • If you get hungry between lunch and dinner, have some fruit or nuts
6–7 P.M.	Dinner Ideas: • Gluten-free pasta with zucchini in tomato sauce • Thai coconut curry with jasmine rice • Lentil soup with roasted vegetables and brown rice • Mushroom and black bean tacos • Buckwheat noodles, stir-fried vegetables, and tofu • Cup of cumin, coriander, and fennel (CCF) tea after dinner
9–10 P.M.	Screens off Meditation, breathing exercise, and/or yoga nidra Journaling and/or reading Mini oil massage for your hands and feet to optimize sleep Lights out!
Important!	Drink 12–16 cups of warm water between meals. This will help flush out those toxins!

a simple swab of our mouth will tell us a lot about our microbial makeup and disease risk.

Ayurveda recommends two simple steps to ensure a healthy oral microbiome: oil pulling and tongue scraping. These habits are important to continue all the time, not just during your reset.

Oil pulling is believed to help with gingivitis, dry mouth, plaque buildup, and bad breath. It can also potentially help with teeth whitening and improve the strength of our jaw muscles, and we know from studies that it can reduce plaque and bacteria in the mouth.[7]

It involves swishing a quarter teaspoon of coconut, sesame, or sunflower oil in the mouth for several minutes, although coconut oil is the most popular due to its antimicrobial, antifungal, and anti-inflammatory properties. Once your mouth becomes full of saliva mixed with the oil, spit it out. I suggest starting out with two minutes of swishing, and increase the time as tolerated. Then brush and floss as normal.

We go to the dentist regularly for our teeth and gums, but we usually neglect the tongue. In Eastern medicine, it's an important aspect of the prevention, diagnosis, and treatment of diseases. Before we had CT scans and MRIs, ancient doctors looked at the tongue to make a diagnosis. A normal tongue is pink with a clear or whitish coating, no teeth marks on the edges, and no major discoloration.

I have seen many tongues in my practice, and no two are alike. In fact, your tongue will look different depending on the time of day or how you feel. Nevertheless, signs of imbalance within different organs include: (1) a thick, white coating, (2) a dry, cracked tongue, (3) bluish or greenish discoloration, and (4) teeth marks on the edges.

Since our tongue is the window into our internal organs, it's important to take good care of it. We need to keep it clean so that it doesn't house bad bacteria. For this reason, both Ayurvedic and Chinese medicine recommend daily tongue scraping. You can buy a metal tongue scraper at most drugstores these days. I suggest scraping it three or four times after you perform oil pulling, and then floss and brush your teeth. It takes just a few seconds, but your oral microbiome will thank you. Even your dentist will be happy, because studies have shown that tongue scraping reduces plaque buildup.[8]

Oil Massage

Abhyanga is a type of Ayurvedic massage that involves the use of warm herbal oils, based on one's dosha, that are massaged into the body with a series of long strokes, kneading, and circular motions. The practice of abhyanga is thought to help promote physical, mental, and emotional well-being by stimulating the body's natural healing abilities.

It is believed to improve circulation, enhance immunity, reduce stress and anxiety, and promote better sleep. Abhyanga is often performed as part of a larger Ayurvedic wellness regimen and is recommended for individuals of all ages and constitutions. It is typically practiced in a warm, quiet, and relaxing environment and is often accompanied by soothing music and aromatherapy to enhance the overall experience.

I often recommend it to my patients, especially for those who struggle with anxiety and insomnia. Applying warm sesame oil or almond oil on one's feet at night can have a calming effect on the body. During the 28-day reset, I encourage doing a full body, warm oil, self-massage daily since it can also help loosen up toxins by improving circulation. If you don't have time for a full-body massage, then feet or face massages are good options and take only a few minutes to perform.

Here are the general steps for self-abhyanga:

1. Choose an oil suitable for your dosha type or any oil that you prefer. Commonly used oils are sesame oil (vata, kapha), coconut oil (pitta), almond oil, or olive oil (all doshas).

2. Warm the oil slightly by placing it in a container and immersing the container in a bowl of hot water. The oil should be comfortably warm but not too hot.

3. Find a warm, quiet, and comfortable space where you can apply the oil. You may also want to place an old towel or cloth on the floor to catch any drips.

4. Start by applying the warm oil to the scalp and massaging it in circular motions. Then move to the face, ears, neck, and shoulders, using gentle strokes. Use long strokes on the limbs and circular motions on the joints. Massage the abdomen and lower back in a clockwise direction.

5. Spend at least three to five minutes on each part of the body to allow the oil to penetrate the skin and nourish the tissues.

6. After massaging the whole body, relax for 15 to 20 minutes to allow the oil to soak in. This is a good time to meditate, journal, or listen to relaxing music. If you have access to a sauna, this might be a good time to use it. Stay warm and relaxed.

7. Rinse off the oil in a warm shower or bath. Avoid a very hot shower, as it can dry your skin. You can also use a mild soap to remove any excess oil.

8. Rest now for a few minutes to allow your body to absorb the benefits of the oil, and you might just sleep like a baby at night. It's also okay to leave the oil on overnight and shower in the morning.

It's important to note that the self-abhyanga technique may vary based on your specific needs and preferences. If you have any medical conditions, consult with your doctor first.

Herbal Therapy

As a part of the reset, I prescribe certain herbal combinations to my patients to facilitate the detoxification process. These herbs have been used for thousands of years to optimize gut health. Recent studies have demonstrated that they can alter our microbiome[9] in a way that optimizes the ratio of good and bad bacteria in the gut. I generally suggest taking two to four tablets or one-half to one teaspoon of *triphala* powder in a cup of hot water at bedtime. Triphala is a combination of three herbs, used for gentle daily detoxification. It is considered to be the king of herbal combinations in Ayurveda. Titrate the dose as needed to attain one to three bowel movements a day during the preparation phase.

Additional herbal combinations that I suggest to my patients include herbs that detox the gut, liver, kidneys, and blood:

- Banyan Botanicals Total Body Cleanse: 2 tablets in the morning
- Banyan Botanicals Blood Cleanse: 2 tablets in the morning

> *Caution: These herbs should not be taken by women while menstruating, pregnant, or breastfeeding. Always consult your doctor before adding any herbs or supplements to your regimen.*

Phase 2: Detoxification

The next seven days will be challenging! Don't be surprised if you dream of hamburgers and milkshakes at night. You might get all sorts of cravings as your body goes through a bit of withdrawal from all the toxins you're about to release.

Think back to a time when you were sick with the flu. While your body was busy fighting the infection, your digestion slowed down. You lost your appetite and ended up eating simple, soothing foods like soups, stews, and fruits. When we're sick, the last thing we want is a steak dinner. Phase 2 is similar, but instead of fighting an infection, your body will dedicate its energy to getting rid of toxins. Your digestive fire will be sluggish, slow, and weak during this time, like cooking with a hot plate instead of a chef's kitchen. So, rather than make a Thanksgiving turkey, you'll stick to simple meals. Eating more than your body can process will only cause indigestion, gas, bloating, and acid reflux.

Diet

	Additional foods to avoid	Reasons	Eat this instead
Nightshades	White potatoes, peppers, eggplant, tomatoes	• Increases inflammation	Zucchini, sweet potato, pumpkin, carrots, asparagus, cooked spinach, peas
FODMAPs	Garlic, onions, mushrooms	• Causes indigestion, bloating	
Leftovers	Food should be consumed within 24 hours of cooking	• Less nutritional value • More gas and bloating • Affects the gut microbiome	Make two servings for the day
Cold foods	Iced beverages, frozen foods	• Diminishes digestive fire • Causes indigestion and acid reflux	Warm foods such as soups and stews
Beans	Chickpeas; beans such as kidney, white, black, pinto, lima, adzuki	• Hard to digest • Causes gas and bloating	Mung beans, lentils (green, black, orange)
Grains	Quinoa, sorghum, amaranth, buckwheat, teff, corn	• Hard to digest • Some grains such as quinoa contain saponins, which are toxic	Rice, oats

In Phase 2, you'll dial back to two meals per day. For each of these, you will stick to one protein, one grain, and one fat. This mono-diet will make it easy for your body to digest the meal, ideally within four hours. The less energy your body spends on digestion, the more it can focus on detoxification.

It's natural to feel hungry part of the time since you're skipping one meal a day. You can satisfy your hunger and aid the detox process by drinking plenty of warm water and herbal teas. Instead of breakfast, you can have 16 ounces of ginger tea with lemon and honey.

Also, please avoid other categories of food that can be hard to digest. None of these foods that you might temporarily avoid are inherently bad for you. Therefore, it is not necessary to avoid them all the time. But during the detox phase, your digestion will be weaker. Since these foods are harder to digest, they can cause inflammation if they aren't metabolized properly. Hence, it is best to avoid until your digestion is optimized and detoxification process is completed.

Don't worry—there are plenty of healthy, delicious foods you can enjoy while you detox. One of my go-to meals during detox is called *khichari*. It's an Indian porridge made with rice, split mung beans, ghee, and spices. As a child, whenever I didn't feel well, I ate it at least a couple of times a week. Instead of chicken soup, it's my favorite comfort food. It's also the first thing I eat when I come home after traveling. It's nourishing and easy to digest. With the right amount of protein, carbs, and fat, it's a balanced meal in and of itself. You can follow the recipe here or find one online. Besides khichari, here are some other meal ideas you can enjoy for either lunch or dinner:

- Fried rice with edamame
- Red lentil coconut curry with pumpkin
- Mung bean soup with zucchini and dill
- Rice noodles with steamed broccoli
- Carrot ginger soup

Khichari Recipe

Serves 2

½ cup basmati rice
½ cup split yellow mung beans
1 tablespoon ghee/clarified butter, or coconut oil if you want to
    keep it vegan
1 bay leaf (optional)
2 to 3 whole cloves or ⅛ teaspoon clove powder
1 small cinnamon stick or ⅛ teaspoon cinnamon powder
½ teaspoon cumin seeds or cumin powder
½ teaspoon turmeric powder
Salt and pepper to taste
Any vegetables such as peas, carrots, pumpkin, or zucchini
    (optional)
Fresh cilantro for garnish (optional)

Soak the rice and mung beans overnight to make them easy to digest. Rinse them well before cooking.

In a 6-quart saucepan, heat the ghee on high. Add the spices and sauté for 1 minute.

Add the rice, mung beans, and vegetables. Sauté for 2 more minutes.

Add 6 cups of water, and bring the mixture to a boil.

Reduce the flame to low/medium and cover, stirring occasionally to avoid burning or sticking. Cook for 30 minutes or until the rice and mung beans are well cooked.

Remove the bay leaf. Garnish with fresh cilantro, if desired. Serve hot.

Lifestyle

During Phase 2, a lot of your energy will go toward detoxification, so again, don't overdo it with exercise. Stick to gentle walking and stretching.

Instead of breaking a sweat through working out, use infrared saunas, steam baths, a heating pad, or just a good, old hot shower. Avoid extreme temperatures, however, and know your limits. Make sure you hydrate well before and after any sauna sessions. This is your chance if you have a bathtub that you've always planned to use but never had the time. Add a few drops of lavender essential oil to your bath, play some soothing music, and pretend you're on a spa vacation.

Sample Daily Routine	
6:00–6:30 A.M.	Rise Start your day by expressing gratitude and setting an intention for the day Oral Care: • Oil pulling with 1/2 teaspoon of coconut or sesame oil • Brush your teeth and floss like your dentist is watching • Tongue scraping Drink 16 ounces of warm water; add lemon if you like A bowel movement should follow soon after
6:30–7:30 A.M.	Meditation Breathing exercises, yoga-based stretches, or a gentle, half-hour walk Body oil massage (abhyanga, a special Indian oil massage, is described on page 187) followed by a 15-minute sauna (infrared, steam, or traditional) or just a hot bath
8–9 A.M.	Breakfast: 16 ounces of ginger tea with lemon and honey
11–12 P.M.	Lunch Ideas: • Fried rice with edamame • Red lentil coconut curry with pumpkin • Khichari stew with split mung beans and rice • Cup of cumin, coriander, and fennel (CCF) tea after lunch
5–6 P.M.	Dinner Ideas: • Mung bean soup with zucchini and dill • Rice noodles with steamed broccoli • Carrot ginger soup • CCF tea after dinner
9–10 P.M.	Screens off Meditation, breathing exercise, yoga nidra Journaling or reading Oil massage for your hands and feet to optimize sleep, if you like Lights out!

As your body relaxes and purges physical and emotional toxins, you're bound to have some exciting revelations. Thoughts, sensations, and emotions might bubble up that have been locked away deep inside. I suggest dedicating more time to reflection and journaling during this week.

Herbal Therapy

During Phase 2, it's time to kick it up a notch with herbs as your ally to flush out toxins. Increase the dose of herbs from Phase 1, and add the following herbs to give you a deeper gut detox.

- Banyan Botanicals Total Body Cleanse: 2 tablets after breakfast and 1 tablet after dinner
- Banyan Botanicals Blood Cleanse: 2 tablets after breakfast and 1 tablet after dinner
- Triphala: 2 tablets before bedtime
- Haritaki: 2 tablets before bedtime

Haritaki is one of the three herbs found in triphala. It is known for its gut-cleansing effect. Hence, during this phase we take more haritaki, in addition to what is found in triphala for additional gut detoxification.

While taking these herbs, you may have more bowel movements than usual. They may also be looser and vary in color and smell. Don't forget to look before you flush! What comes out of your body tells you a lot about what's happening inside. You might be shocked to see what comes out of you, even when eating a very simple diet. What you're purging are toxins from all the undigested foods that have accumulated over time. They are finally being mobilized so that you can get rid of them instead of allowing them to take root in your body and lead to diseases.

Remember to hydrate well with warm water throughout the day!

Phase 3: Reintroduction

Now that you have peed, pooped, and sweated out the toxins, you might feel lighter. The most important takeaway from this phase is how much better you can feel when you do less. It's a crucial lesson to realize you can deal with hunger pangs, food cravings, and temptations. Now you know that you can conquer them all and feel better than you ever have. Regaining control of what you choose to put in your body is a reward in itself.

Therefore, instead of rushing back to your usual diet and lifestyle, it's important to take it one step at a time. After the detox, your body is like a clean slate, and going right back to your usual can undo your hard work way too fast. Over the next week, you'll slowly add back more foods and activity.

Be gentle, mindful, and intentional as you get back to your daily routine. We are usually used to running around like mad hares. Instead, be slow and steady like the tortoise. We all know who wins in the end.

Diet

The first thing you'll reintroduce is breakfast. Start with fresh fruit or green juice for two days, and then add grains. Here are some seasonal recommendations for easy-to-digest breakfasts that are perfect for the reintroduction phase:

Summer/Spring:

- Bowl of seasonal fresh fruits
- Fresh-pressed juice with celery, cucumber, apple, and ginger, served at room temperature
- Overnight oats with chia seeds, dried apricots, and honey, served at room temperature

Winter/Fall:

- Hot water with ginger, lemon, cinnamon, and honey
- Congee
- Steel-cut oatmeal with coconut sugar, cinnamon, and raisins. Add extra water to give the oatmeal a soupy consistency, and avoid adding nuts since they can be a bit heavy to digest.

Besides adding breakfast back into your diet, you will also reintroduce grains, vegetables, and legumes that you eliminated during the detox. You will add foods in order of how easy they are to process as listed in the table below.

Continue to avoid cold foods and beverages while minimizing leftovers. You can now eat foods within 48 hours of cooking them instead of 24 hours.

Order of Food Reintroduction	
Nightshades	White potatoes, peppers, eggplant, tomatoes
FODMAPs	Garlic, onions, mushrooms
Beans	Chickpeas; beans such as kidney, white, black, pinto, lima, adzuki, or any other beans you avoided
Grains	Quinoa, sorghum, amaranth, buckwheat, teff, corn or any other grains you avoided

As you add foods back into your diet, you may notice that some cause digestive discomfort. You may also experience other symptoms, such as brain fog, joint pain, and sluggishness with certain foods. If you identify such triggers, you should avoid the foods that might have led to them for another week as you continue to add more agreeable foods. This type of elimination diet helps identify hidden triggers of inflammation in the body.

Lifestyle

Slowly increase your activity level with slightly more strenuous workouts. Always listen to your body, however, and see how you feel. There's no need to push yourself beyond what's comfortable.

Within a few days, some people can get back to their usual diet and activity level, while others take a bit longer. Be patient with yourself.

Herbs

It's time to ease off the detox herbs as you shift gears from detox to rejuvenation. You can stop the Banyan Botanical Total Body Cleanse, Total Blood Cleanse, and haritaki at this point. Please continue taking two tablets of triphala before bedtime.

Phase 4: Rejuvenation

After all your hard work during Phases 1, 2, and 3, it's time to reap the rewards. So far, you've slowed down your metabolism during Phase 1, detoxed in Phase 2, and ramped back up again in Phase 3. Everything you've done is to optimize your metabolism. Now your body is far more receptive to rejuvenation without toxins getting in the way.

The rejuvenation phase will continue for the next three to six months. Some benefits of the 28-day reset manifest even after several months, so pay close attention. The following are some of the benefits you may notice after the 28 days:

- Stronger immune system
- Decrease in inflammation
- More acute senses: hearing, taste, vision, touch, and smell
- Improved concentration and memory
- Lower stress and anxiety
- Boost in energy and libido

- Improved muscle recovery time, less joint stiffness
- More regular and complete bowel movements
- Improved skin complexion
- Stronger, faster-growing hair and nails

Since the rejuvenation phase continues for months in the background, it's helpful to include certain "positive" energy foods in your diet, which can enhance the process. These include nuts, seeds, sprouted legumes and grains, fresh fruits and vegetables, and certain spices.

For the next week, however, your diet, lifestyle, and daily routine will be the same as in Phase 1. The central part of rejuvenation is adding certain herbs to enhance the process so that you can achieve even better results. In Ayurveda, all the rejuvenating herbs are combined into a delicious jam called *chyavanprash*. It contains more than 30 different herbs and spices that work seamlessly together. These herbs are far more effective when taken after a detox.

For the next week, you will take one teaspoon of Banyan Botanicals Chyavanprash twice a day with meals. After that, you will take one teaspoon once a day for the next three months.

You will also continue taking two tablets of triphala at bedtime for the next three months. This is something I suggest most of my patients take for a lifetime!

AFTER 28 DAYS . . .

Bravo! Now that you've completed the reset, take a moment to reflect on your journey. You have purged not only physical but also emotional toxins that you were harboring for a long time. Now you have a powerful tool in your toolbox with the 28-day reset at your disposal. Do it at least once a year to bring your body back into balance. This is indeed the ancient recipe for staying young, increasing vitality, and preventing diseases for years to come.

FREQUENTLY ASKED QUESTIONS

What if I don't have 28 days, but I need a quick reset?
Here's a quick guide to a shorter regimen to fit your needs. I always encourage my patients to incorporate a shorter regimen anytime they need to reset their metabolism.

Reset Duration	3 days	1 week	10 days
Phase 1: Preparation	1 day	2 days	3 days
Phase 2: Detoxification	1 day	3 days	4 days
Phase 3: Reintroduction	1 day	2 days	3 days
Phase 4: Rejuvenation	1 week	2 weeks	3 weeks

I don't think I can eat just twice a day. What if I get hungry?
Hunger is uncomfortable, but I assure you that your body is better equipped to deal with hunger than overeating. I highly recommend drinking ginger, lemon, and honey tea to help with hunger pangs or mental/emotional cravings. This will fill your stomach, improve your metabolism, and help you stick to the 28-day plan.

I'm not used to cooking. What do I do?
Fortunately, there are excellent meal delivery services that you can use to make your life easier. Plant-based meal delivery service options include Sunbasket, Purple Carrot, Daily Harvest, Mosaic, Green Chef, and Sakara. Also, look for local plant-based, healthy restaurants.

I have many food allergies and intolerances. How can I customize my diet for the 28-day reset?
First, identify a gluten-free grain, plant-based protein, and plant-based fat that agree with you. These will compose the mono-diet that you can use for Phase 2. During Phases 1 and 3, you will have more options to include foods that don't bother you. When you're in doubt, I highly recommend working with a

knowledgeable nutritionist or a registered dietitian who can further customize your diet.

I'm not familiar with the herbs. Where can I buy them?
Most of the herbs I mentioned can be easily found at a health food store, or you can find them online to be shipped almost anywhere.

I don't like the taste of the herbs. Are there any alternatives?
Medicines sometimes taste like medicine. They don't come in fruit flavors. I don't enjoy taking herbs that taste like dirt either, but they work best when taken in their natural form, so pinch your nose and do it for your body.

CHAPTER 10

THE 20-MINUTE DAILY RITUAL

After completing the 28-day reset, your body has shifted gears to rejuvenate itself—a process that will continue for several months. At the end of the reset, you have a choice to make. Do you want to enhance and prolong the effect of the reset by dedicating a few minutes to your well-being daily, or do you want to let toxins accumulate until the next time you do a reset?

The choice is straightforward, in my opinion. Vacations to Italy aside, if I can dedicate 20 minutes daily to continue reaping the benefits of the reset, I'll do it. This small investment will pay off in the long run by optimizing your health and preventing diseases. It's also much easier to stick to a ritual if you do it every day. After all, we're creatures of habit.

These habits are also easy to assimilate into your day without a big-time commitment. They may seem insignificant at first, but trust me, they're foundational. The reason I focus on these small practices is that they set the tone for everything else you do in your day. They'll have an impact on all four pillars of intentional health: diet, sleep, exercise, and stress management. If you want the biggest bang for your buck from the food you eat, your exercise regimen, and your sleep, start with a strong foundation.

YOUR DAILY RITUAL

The components of the daily ritual are nothing new. You've already learned about them in previous chapters and practiced them for 28 days. Now it's simply time to implement them on a regular basis.

Let's get started with making your daily routine. If you need more information, refer to the circadian rhythm chapter. Fill in the following to establish a blueprint for your day:

Wake-up time: _____
Exercise: _____
Breakfast: _____
Lunch: _____
Dinner: _____
Bedtime: _____

Let's review what the 20-minute daily ritual entails.

As soon as you wake up, you may be accustomed to looking at your phone and scrolling through e-mails or the news. I can't think of a better way to raise your cortisol and alter your circadian rhythm—two things you *don't* want. Instead, take just two minutes to set an intention while taking deep, diaphragmatic breaths. This will set a more positive tone for your day.

The deep breathing activates your vagus nerve, reduces cortisol, and gets you out of the fight-or-flight response (especially on a Monday morning). By setting a positive intention and visualizing how you want your day to manifest, you can shape your thoughts and actions, consciously and unconsciously, for the next 24 hours and beyond. Doesn't this sound like a much better way to start the day? The e-mails and news can wait a couple of minutes; they aren't going anywhere.

The next stop is the kitchen—not for a muffin or bagel, but for a tall glass of warm water. As we reviewed earlier, warm water stimulates your gastrocolic reflex and hydrates you first thing in the morning. Hopefully, a bowel movement will follow soon after. Taking the trash and toxins out of your body in the morning on

20-Minute Daily Routine		
Activity	Time	Reasons
Wake up	7 A.M.	Syncing your circadian rhythm
Set a positive intention for the day / Deep breathing	2 minutes	Visualization and reducing cortisol
Glass of warm water on an empty stomach	2 minutes	Gut health and detox by promoting health Regular bowel movement
Oral care, including oil pulling and tongue scraping	3 minutes	Optimizing your oral and gut microbiome Maintaining dental health
Exercise	7:30 A.M. or 5:30 P.M.	Enhancing physical strength and flexibility
Mindful eating Deep breathing for 1 minute prior to meals	3 minutes	Activating the rest-and-digest system
Breakfast	9 A.M.	Strengthening your digestive fire with regular mealtimes
Lunch	1 P.M.	
Dinner	6 P.M.	
Deep breathing / Journaling / Guided imagery / Progressive muscle relaxation	10 minutes	Activating your vagus nerve Optimizing the mind-body connection Enhancing sleep quality
Bedtime	10 P.M.	Syncing circadian rhythm

a regular basis is one of the most important things you can do to ensure your gut health.

During your annual physical, your doctor may ask you about preventative exams, such as a mammogram or colonoscopy. In addition to those screening exams, I also ask my patients about their last visit to the dentist. Some of my patients would rather have a colonoscopy than have their teeth and gums examined.

However, based on what you've learned, oral health and the oral microbiome are very important for overall health.

To support them, it makes sense to continue oil pulling and tongue scraping. I recommend doing these daily. If you frequent the dentist's office more than you'd like due to tooth and gum problems, stick to this daily practice. They just might reduce your dentist visits. Plus, they'll ensure fresher breath and less plaque.

Once you've finished your morning routine and are carrying on with your busy day, check in with yourself often. One of the best times to stop and smell the roses is around your mealtimes. We're so accustomed to eating on the go or while answering e-mails or watching television that we forget to practice mindful eating, which optimizes digestion, activates the vagus nerve, and gets us out of stress mode into rest-and-digest mode. All you have to do is breathe!

Take a minute before you eat to become fully present. Take a few deep breaths to start, and then pay close attention to the texture, taste, and temperature of the food. Engage all your senses. This will ensure that you produce ample gastric juices and allow for enough time to chew and digest. Another benefit of eating mindfully is that you'll actually enjoy your food and be less likely to overeat. Not to mention, you are more likely to avoid unsavory gastrointestinal symptoms such as acid reflux, gas, and bloating. Bon appétit!

When you're done with your busy day, you can finally look forward to unwinding. After dinner, you may spend some time with your family, watch a TV show, or get cozy with a book. However you choose to unwind, make sure you spare at least 10 minutes to get your mind and body ready for sleep. What we do right before bed can have a significant impact on the quality and quantity of our slumber. Small things like blue-light exposure, alcohol, and/or eating a late dinner can get in the way of good sleep.

Invest some time before bed to engage in a relaxation activity. You can choose to simply lie in bed with your eyes closed as you practice deep breathing, or you can listen to a guided meditation. You may want to write in your journal or perform progressive muscle relaxation. Just 10 minutes can activate your vagus nerve and change your brain waves to invite restful sleep.

Who knew that you could optimize your mind-body connection, add positivity, support your microbiome and digestive fire, enhance detox, and activate your vagus nerve by simply dedicating 20 minutes per day to it? Make it a routine and stick to it (even during those pasta-filled vacations in Italy). It's an investment worth making for your health for years to come.

OPTIMAL HEALTH

As the book comes to an end, I want to remind you once again that we are all superhumans. We are born with a body that has the intelligence of millions of years of evolution. It knows how to overcome adversities by adapting and evolving. We are in control of this masterful machinery, which can help us live well past 100 years—even 185 years!

Anytime we are out of balance, our body knows how to bring us back to health. Diseases take root when we're working against our normal physiologic processes. The ancient secrets have taught us what optimal health looks like and what we can do to maintain it. Think of them as a user manual for our body. Now that you know the fundamentals of how to keep this body running like a well-oiled machine, no more patching things up. Instead, you can work with your body and bring it back to balance whenever you want.

According to ancient wisdom, each living being has the universal life force, which I mentioned earlier is also known as *prana* or *qi* (*chi*), flowing through them. When it flows freely, unobstructed, it manifests itself as vitality. It has the power to heal and regenerate every cell in our body. This is optimal health. With ancient knowledge on our side, we can now unlock the secret of living a life full of vitality, which is much more than just the absence of diseases. Our human destiny is to thrive, not just survive. The secrets revealed in this book can help us do so by unlocking our body's true potential.

You have all the knowledge you need to embark on your intentional health journey. Knowledge is power when it is actionable. Understanding how to make your body work optimally and how to bring it back to balance is the key to longevity and preventing diseases. Now you can take charge of your health with ancient wisdom as your guide.

ENDNOTES

Introduction

1. "Constitution of the World Health Organization," World Health Organization, https://www.who.int/about/governance/constitution.

2. Mayo Clinic Staff, "Stem Cells: What They Are and What They Do," Mayo Clinic, March 19, 2022, accessed August 13, 2022, https://www.mayoclinic.org/tests-procedures/bone-marrow-transplant/in-depth/stem-cells/art-20048117.

3. P. Mistriotis and S. T. Andreadis, "Hair Follicle: A Novel Source of Multipotent Stem Cells for Tissue Engineering and Regenerative Medicine," *Tissue Engineering Part B: Reviews* 19, no. 4, (2013): 265–78, https://doi.org/10.1089/ten.TEB.2012.0422.

4. A. W. Duncan, C. Dorrell, and M. Grompe, "Stem Cells and Liver Regeneration," *Gastroenterology* 137, no. 2 (2009): 466–81, https://doi.org/10.1053/j.gastro.2009.05.044.

5. "Stem Cell Transplants in Cancer Treatment," National Cancer Institute, April 29, 2015, accessed August 13, 2022, https://www.cancer.gov/about-cancer/treatment/types/stem-cell-transplant.

6. National Center for Health Statistics, "Leading Causes of Death," Centers for Disease and Control and Prevention, January 13, 2022, accessed August 13, 2022, https://www.cdc.gov/nchs/fastats/leading-causes-of-death.htm.

Chapter 1

1. Thinnes-Elker et al., "Intention Concepts and Brain-Machine Interfacing," *Frontiers in Psychology* 3 (2012): 455, https://doi.org/10.3389/fpsyg.2012.00455.

2. E. Plys and O. Desrichard, "Associations between Positive and Negative Affect and the Way People Perceive Their Health Goals," *Frontiers in Psychology* 11 (2020): 334, https://doi.org/10.3389/fpsyg.2020.00334.

3. Yanek et al., "Effect of Positive Well-Being on Incidence of Symptomatic Coronary Artery Disease," *American Journal of Cardiology* 112, no. 8 (2013): 1120–5, https://doi.org/10.1016/j.amjcard.2013.05.055.

4. Long et al., "The Role of Hope in Subsequent Health and Well-Being for Older Adults: An Outcome-Wide Longitudinal Approach," *Global Epidemiology* 2 (2020): 100018, https://doi.org/10.1016/j.gloepi.2020.100018.

5. A. Vaish, T. Grossmann, and A. Woodward, "Not All Emotions Are Created Equal: The Negativity Bias in Social-Emotional Development." *Psychological Bulletin* 134, no. 3 (2008): 383–403, https://doi.org/10.1037/0033-2909.134.3.383.

6. L. G. Kiken and N. J. Shook, "Looking Up: Mindfulness Increases Positive Judgments and Reduces Negativity Bias," *Social Psychological and Personality Science* 2, no. 4 (2011): 425–31, https://doi.org/10.1177/1948550610396585.

Chapter 2

1. Li et al., "A New Perspective for Parkinson's Disease: Circadian Rhythm," *Neuroscience Bulletin* 33, no. 1 (2017): 62–72, https://doi.org/10.1007/s12264 -016-0089-7.

2. A. W. C. Man, H. Li, and N. Xia, "Circadian Rhythm: Potential Therapeutic Target for Atherosclerosis and Thrombosis," *International Journal of Molecular Sciences* 22, no. 2 (2021): 676, https://doi.org/10.3390/ijms22020676.

3. Rácz et al., "Links between the Circadian Rhythm, Obesity and the Microbiome," *Physiological Research* 67, Suppl 3 (2018): S409–S420, https:// doi.org/10.33549/physiolres.934020.

4. O. Çalıyurt, "Role of Chronobiology as a Transdisciplinary Field of Research: Its Applications in Treating Mood Disorders," *Balkan Medical Journal* 34, no. 6 (2017):514–21, https://doi.org/10.4274/balkanmedj.2017.1280.

5. G. Sulli, M. T. Y. Lam, and S. Panda, "Interplay between Circadian Clock and Cancer: New Frontiers for Cancer Treatment," *Trends Cancer* 5, no. 8 (2019): 475–94, https://doi.org/10.1016/j.trecan.2019.07.002.

6. Gina Kolata, "2017 Nobel Prize in Medicine Goes to 3 Americans for Body Clock Studies," *New York Times*, October 2, 2017, accessed July 7, 2022.

7. K. Bates and E. D. Herzog, "Maternal-Fetal Circadian Communication during Pregnancy," *Frontiers in Endocrinology* 11 (2020): 198, https://doi.org/10.3389/ fendo.2020.00198.

8. R. Orozco-Solis and L. Aguilar-Arnal, "Circadian Regulation of Immunity through Epigenetic Mechanisms," *Frontiers in Cellular Infection Microbiology* 10 (2020): 96, https://doi.org/10.3389/fcimb.2020.00096.

9. Xu et al., "The Circadian Clock and Inflammation: A New Insight," *Clinica Chimica Acta* 512 (2021): 12–7, https://doi.org/10.1016/j.cca.2020.11.011.

10. Sato et al., "Possible Contribution of Chronobiology to Cardiovascular Health," *Frontiers in Physiology* 4 (2014): 409, https://doi.org/10.3389/fphys .2013.00409.

11. Rahman et al., "Characterizing the Temporal Dynamics of Melatonin and Cortisol Changes in Response to Nocturnal Light Exposure," *Scientific Reports* 9, no. 1 (2019): 19720, https://doi.org/10.1038/s41598-019-54806-7.

12. M. H. Smolensky, L. L. Sackett-Lundeen, and F. Portaluppi, "Nocturnal Light Pollution and Underexposure to Daytime Sunlight: Complementary Mechanisms of Circadian Disruption and Related Diseases," *Chronobiology International* 32, no. 8 (2015): 1029–48, https://doi.org/10.3109/07420528.20 15.1072002.

13. Chao et al., "Stress, Cortisol, and Other Appetite-Related Hormones: Prospective Prediction of 6-Month Changes in Food Cravings and Weight," *Obesity (Silver Spring)* 25, no. 4 (2017): 713–20, https://doi.org/10.1002 /oby.21790.

14. Q. Xiao, M. Garaulet, and F. A. J. L. Scheer, "Meal Timing and Obesity: Interactions with Macronutrient Intake and Chronotype," *International Journal of Obesity (London)* 43, no. 9 (2019): 1701–11, https://doi.org/10.1038/s41366-018-0284-x.

15. Deshmukh-Taskar et al., "The Relationship of Breakfast Skipping and Type of Breakfast Consumed with Overweight/Obesity, Abdominal Obesity, Other Cardiometabolic Risk Factors and the Metabolic Syndrome in Young Adults. The National Health and Nutrition Examination Survey (NHANES): 1999–2006," *Public Health Nutrition* 16, no. 11 (2013): 2073–82, https://doi.org/10.1017/S1368980012004296.

16. Garaulet et al., "Timing of Food Intake Predicts Weight Loss Effectiveness." *International Journal of Obesity (London)* 37, no. 4 (2013): 604–11, https://doi.org/10.1038/ijo.2012.229.

17. Baron et al., "Contribution of Evening Macronutrient Intake to Total Caloric Intake and Body Mass Index," *Appetite* 60, no. 1 (2013): 246–51, https://doi.org/10.1016/j.appet.2012.09.026.

18. E. Manzano, "Too Much or Too Little Sleep Triggers Constipation," MIMS Gastroenterology, June 17, 2020, accessed July 7, 2022, https://specialty.mims.com/topic/too-much-or-too-little-sleep-triggers-constipation-#:~:text=%E2%80%9COr%2C%20it%20may%20also%20be,sleep%20on%20constipation%2C%20said%20Adejumo.

19. K. Rodriguez, "How to Hack Your Brain for Creative Ideas Before You Even Get Out of Bed," *Fast Company*, August 12, 2016, accessed July 7, 2022, https://www.fastcompany.com/3062746/how-to-hack-your-brain-for-creative-ideas-before-you-even-get-out-.

20. Cedars-Sinai Medical Center, "When Memory-Related Neurons Fire in Sync with Certain Brain Waves, Memories Last," *ScienceDaily*, March 28, 2010, accessed July 7, 2022, https://www.sciencedaily.com/releases/2010/03/100324142115.htm.

21. S. D. Youngstedt, J. A. Elliott, and D. F. Kripke, "Human Circadian Phase-Response Curves for Exercise," *The Journal of Physiology* 597, no. 8 (2019): 2253–68, https://doi.org/10.1113/JP276943.

22. Fairbrother et al., "Effects of Exercise Timing on Sleep Architecture and Nocturnal Blood Pressure in Prehypertensives," *Vascular Health and Risk Management* 10 (2014): 691–8, https://doi.org/10.2147/VHRM.S73688.

23. The Redbooth Team. "Everybody's Working for the Weekend, But When Do You Actually Get Work Done?" *Redbooth*, November 15, 2017, accessed July 7, 2022, https://redbooth.com/blog/your-most-productive-time.

24. Harvard Health Publishing Staff, "Intermittent Fasting: The Positive News Continues," Harvard Medical School, February 28, 2021, accessed July 7, 2022, https://www.health.harvard.edu/blog/intermittent-fasting-surprising-update-2018062914156.

25. A. Paoli, "Ketogenic Diet for Obesity: Friend or Foe?" *International Journal of Environmental Research Public Health* 11, no. 2 (2014): 2092–107, https://doi.org/10.3390/ijerph110202092.

26. National Geographic Society, "Light Pollution," *National Geographic*, last updated June 2, 2022, accessed July 7, 2022, https://education.national geographic.org/resource/light-pollution.

27. Ishizawa et al., "Effects of Pre-Bedtime Blue-Light Exposure on Ratio of Deep Sleep in Healthy Young Men," *Sleep Medicine* 84 (2021): 303–7, https://doi .org/10.1016/j.sleep.2021.05.046.

28. Park et al., "Association of Exposure to Artificial Light at Night While Sleeping with Risk of Obesity in Women," *JAMA Internal Medicine* 179, no. 8 (2019): 1061–71, https://doi.org/10.1001/jamainternmed.2019.0571.

29. Hester et al., "Evening Wear of Blue-Blocking Glasses for Sleep and Mood Disorders: A Systematic Review," *Chronobiology International* 38, no. 10 (2021): 1375–83, https://doi.org/10.1080/07420528.2021.1930029.

30. Merikanto et al., "Associations of Chronotype and Sleep with Cardiovascular Diseases and Type 2 Diabetes," *Chronobiology International* 30, no. 4 (2013): 470–7, https://doi.org/10.3109/07420528.2012.741171.

31. M. Paul, "Night Owls at Risk for Weight Gain," Northwestern University, May 4, 2011, accessed July 7, 2022, https://www.northwestern.edu/news center/stories/2011/05/night-owls-weight-gain.html.

32. K. L. Knutson and M. von Schantz, "Associations between Chronotype, Morbidity and Mortality in the UK Biobank Cohort," *Chronobiology International* 35, no. 8 (2018): 1045–53, https://doi.org/10.1080/07420528.2018.1454458.

Chapter 3

1. J. A. Foster, G. B. Baker, and S. M. Dursun, "The Relationship between the Gut Microbiome-Immune System-Brain Axis and Major Depressive Disorder," *Frontiers in Neurology* 12 (2021): 721126, https://doi.org/10.3389/fneur.2021.721126.

2. Li et al., "The Role of Microbiome in Insomnia, Circadian Disturbance and Depression," *Frontiers in Psychiatry* 9 (2018): 669, https://doi.org/10.3389 /fpsyt.2018.00669.

3. F. Bishehsari, R. M. Voigt, and A. Keshavarzian, "Circadian Rhythms and the Gut Microbiota: From the Metabolic Syndrome to Cancer," *Nature Reviews Endocrinology* 16 (2020): 731–9, https://doi.org/10.1038/s41574-020-00427-4.

4. Lambeth et al., "Composition, Diversity and Abundance of Gut Microbiome in Prediabetes and Type 2 Diabetes," *Journal of Diabetes and Obesity* 2, no. 3 (2015): 1–7, https://doi.org/10.15436/2376-0949.15.031.

5. Torres-Fuentes et al., "The Microbiota-Gut-Brain Axis in Obesity," *The Lancet Gastroenterology Hepatology* 2, no. 10 (2017): 747–56, https://doi.org/10.1016 /S2468-1253(17)30147-4.

6. M. Witkowski, T. L. Weeks, and S. L. Hazen, "Gut Microbiota and Cardiovascular Disease," *Circulation Research* 127, no. 4 (2020): 553–70, https://doi.org/10.1161/CIRCRESAHA.120.316242.

7. Mentella et al., "Nutrition, IBD and Gut Microbiota: A Review," *Nutrients* 12, no. 4 (2020): 944, https://doi.org/10.3390/nu12040944.

8. Pecora et al., "Gut Microbiota in Celiac Disease: Is There Any Role for Probiotics?" *Frontiers in Immunology* 11 (2020): 957, https://doi.org/10.3389/fimmu.2020.00957.

9. M. Reiger, V. Schwierzeck, and C. Traidl-Hoffmann, "Atopisches Ekzem und Mikrobiom [Atopic Eczema and Microbiome]," *Hautarzt* 70, no. 6 (2019): 407–15, https://doi.org/10.1007/s00105-019-4424-6.

10. Myers et al., "The Gut Microbiome in Psoriasis and Psoriatic Arthritis," *Best Practice and Research in Clinical Rheumatology* 33, no. 6 (2019): 101494, https://doi.org/10.1016/j.berh.2020.101494.

11. Cryan et al., "The Gut Microbiome in Neurological Disorders," *The Lancet Neurology* 19, no. 2 (2020): 179–94, https://doi.org/10.1016/1474-4422(19)30356-4.

12. Mangiola et al., "Gut Microbiota in Autism and Mood Disorders," *World Journal of Gastroenterology* 22, no. 1 (2016): 361–8, https://doi.org/10.3748/wjg.v22.i1.361.

13. Vighi et al., "Allergy and the gastrointestinal system," *Clin Exp Immunol* 153, Suppl 1(2008): 3–6, https://doi.org/10.1111/j.1365-2249.2008.03713.x.

14. C. Willyard, "What Do Worms Have to Do with Asthma?" *Science*, February 20, 2011, accessed July 9, 2022, https://www.science.org/content/article/what-do-worms-have-do-asthma.

15. Tang et al., "Administration of a Probiotic with Peanut Oral Immunotherapy: A Randomized Trial," *The Journal of Allergy and Clinical Immunology* 135, no. 3 (2015): 737–44.e8, https://doi.org/10.1016/j.jaci.2014.11.034.

16. Gupta et al., "Prevalence and Severity of Food Allergies Among US Adults," *JAMA Network Open* 2, no. 1 (2019): e185630, https://doi.org/10.1001/jamanetworkopen.2018.5630.

17. Allaire et al., "Health-Related Quality of Life among U.S. Adults with and without Food Allergies," *The Journal of the Academy of Nutrition and Dietetics* 121, no. 9, suppl (2021): A25, https://doi.org/10.1016/j.jand.2021.06.059.

18. A. Sutton, "Could a Hidden Allergy Be Causing Your Migraines?" *Harvard University Science in the News*, May 1, 2013, accessed July 9, 2022, https://sitn.hms.harvard.edu/flash/2013/could-a-hidden-allergy-be-causing-your-migraines/.

19. Robert H. Loblay and Anne R. Swain, "The Role of Food Intolerance in Chronic Fatigue Syndrome," in *The Clinical and Scientific Basis of Myalgic Encephalomyelitis Chronic Fatigue Syndrome*, B.M. Hyde, J. Goldstein, and P. Levine, Editors. 1992, The Nightingale Research Foundation: Ottawa. 521–538. https://www.slhd.nsw.gov.au/rpa/Allergy/research/RoleOfFoodIntoleranceInCFS.pdf.

20. "MRT 176, MRT® Food & Chemical Profiles," Oxford Biomedical Technologies, accessed July 9, 2022, https://www.nowleap.com/test-profiles/.

21. J. F. Geiselman, "The Clinical Use of IgG Food Sensitivity Testing with Migraine Headache Patients: A Literature Review," *Current Pain and Headache Reports* 23, no. 11 (2019): 79, https://doi.org/10.1007/s11916-019-0819-4.

22. Thaiss et al., "The Microbiome and Innate Immunity," *Nature* 535 (2016): 65–74, https://doi.org/10.1038/nature18847.

23. Xu et al., "The Dynamic Interplay between the Gut Microbiota and Autoimmune Diseases," *Journal of Immunology Research* (2019): 7546047, https://doi.org/10.1155/2019/7546047.

24. Vangay et al., "Antibiotics, Pediatric Dysbiosis, and Disease," *Cell & Host Microbe* 17, no. 5 (2015): 553–64, https://doi.org/10.1016/j.chom.2015.04.006.

25. M. F. Khan and H. Wang, "Environmental Exposures and Autoimmune Diseases: Contribution of Gut Microbiome," *Frontiers in Immunology* 10 (2020): 3094, https://doi.org/10.3389/fimmu.2019.03094.

26. National Center for Chronic Disease Prevention and Health Promotion, "Inflammatory Bowel Disease, Data and Statistics," Centers for Disease Control and Prevention, last reviewed April 14, 2022, accessed July 9, 2022, https://www.cdc.gov/ibd/data-statistics.htm.

27. Schneider et al., "The Breast Cancer Epidemic: 10 Facts," *The Linacre Quarterly* 81, no. 3 (2014): 244–77, https://doi.org/10.1179/2050854914Y.0000000027.

28. "Breast Cancer Facts and Statistics," BreastCancer.org, last updated March 10, 2022, accessed July 9, 2022, https://www.breastcancer.org/facts-statistics.

29. C. Kresser, "The Gut-Hormone Connection: How Gut Microbes Influence Estrogen Levels," Kresser Institute, November 15, 2017, accessed July 9, 2022, https://kresserinstitute.com/gut-hormone-connection-gut-microbes -influence-estrogen-levels/.

30. B. S. Reddy, J. H. Weisburger, and E. L. Wynder, "Fecal Bacterial Beta-Glucuronidase: Control by Diet," *Science* 183, no. 4123 (1974): 416–7, https://doi.org/10.1126/science.183.4123.416.

31. Poutahidis et al., "Probiotic Microbes Sustain Youthful Serum Testosterone Levels and Testicular Size in Aging Mice," *PLOS ONE* 9, no. 1 (2014): e84877, https://doi.org/10.1371/journal.pone.0084877.

32. J. Chen and L. Vitetta, "Butyrate in Inflammatory Bowel Disease Therapy," *Gastroenterology* 158, no. 5 (2020): 1511, https://doi.org/10.1053/j.gastro .2019.08.064.

33. "Medical Cannabis," Crohn's & Colitis Foundation, accessed July 9, 2022, https://www.crohnscolitisfoundation.org/complementary-medicine /medical-cannabis.

34. N. Shtraizent, Ph.D., "Acupuncture in Inflammatory Bowel Disease," Crohn's & Colitis Foundation, June 18, 2019, accessed July 9, 2022, https://www .crohnscolitisfoundation.org/blog/acupuncture-inflammatory-bowel-disease.

35. Ramirez et al., "Antibiotics as Major Disruptors of Gut Microbiota," *Frontiers in Cellular and Infection Microbiology* 10 (2020): 572912, https://doi.org /10.3389/fcimb.2020.572912.

36. "CDC: 1 in 3 Antibiotic Prescriptions Unnecessary," Centers for Disease Control and Prevention, May 3, 2016, accessed July 9, 2022, https://www .cdc.gov/media/releases/2016/p0503-unnecessary-prescriptions.html.

37. B. Rodgers, K. Kirley, and A. Mounsey, "PURLs: Prescribing an Antibiotic? Pair It with Probiotics," *The Journal of Family Practice* 62, no. 3 (2013): 148–50.

38. Yuan et al., "Gut Microbiota: An Underestimated and Unintended Recipient for Pesticide-Induced Toxicity," *Chemosphere* 227 (2019): 425–34, https://doi .org/10.1016/j.chemosphere.2019.04.088.

39. M. Zhou and J. Zhao, "A Review on the Health Effects of Pesticides Based on Host Gut Microbiome and Metabolomics," *Frontiers in Molecular Biosciences* 8 (2021): 632955, https://doi.org/10.3389/fmolb.2021.632955.

40. "Dirty Dozen™: EWG's 2023 Shopper's Guide to Pesticides in Produce™," Environmental Working Group, accessed March 27, 2023, https://www.ewg .org/foodnews/dirty-dozen.php.

41. Bøhn et al., "Compositional Differences in Soybeans on the Market: Glyphosate Accumulates in Roundup Ready GM Soybeans," *Food Chemistry* 153 (2014): 207–15, https://doi.org/10.1016/j.foodchem.2013.12.054.

42. National Institute of Standards and Technology, "Researchers Advance Efforts to Accurately Measure Glyphosate Pesticide in Oats," *Phys.org*, November 2, 2020, accessed July 9, 2022, https://phys.org/news/2020-11-advance-efforts -accurately-glyphosate-pesticide.html#:~:text=Oats%20tend%20to%20 have%20a,to%20co%2Dauthor%20Justine%20Cruz.

43. "Roundup for Breakfast, Part 2: In New Tests, Weed Killer Found in All Kids' Cereals Sampled," Environmental Working Group, October 24, 2018, accessed July 9, 2022, https://www.ewg.org/news-insights/news-release/2018 /10/roundup-breakfast-part-2-new-tests-weed-killer-found-all-kids.

44. C. Roberts, "An Easy Way to Remove Pesticides," *Consumer Reports*, October 25, 2017, accessed July 9, 2022, https://www.consumerreports.org /pesticides-herbicides/easy-way-to-remove-pesticides-a3616455263/.

45. A. Zander and M. Bunning, "Guide to Washing Fresh Produce," Colorado State University Extension Fact Sheet No. 9.380, accessed July 9, 2022, https://www.nifa.usda.gov/sites/default/files/resource/Guide%20to%20 Washing%20Fresh%20Produce508.pdf.

46. Naimi et al., "Direct Impact of Commonly Used Dietary Emulsifiers on Human Gut Microbiota," *Microbiome* 9, no. 1 (2021): 66, https://doi .org/10.1186/s40168-020-00996-6.

47. "Tartrazine," ScienceDirect, accessed July 9, 2022, https://www.sciencedirect .com/topics/agricultural-and-biological-sciences/tartrazine.

48. Sonuga-Barke et al., "Nonpharmacological Interventions for ADHD: Systematic Review and Meta-Analyses of Randomized Controlled Trials of Dietary And Psychological Treatments," *The American Journal of Psychiatry* 170, no. 3 (2013): 275–89, https://doi.org/10.1176/appi.ajp.2012.12070991.

49. Sarah Kobylewski and Michael F. Jacobson, *Food Dyes: A Rainbow of Risks* (Washington, DC: Center for Science in the Public Interest, 2010).

50. C. Potera, "The Artificial Food Dye Blues," *Environmental Health Perspectives* 118, no. 10 (2010): A428, https://doi.org/10.1289/ehp.118-a428.

51. M. D. Pang, G. H. Goossens, and E. E. Blaak, "The Impact of Artificial Sweeteners on Body Weight Control and Glucose Homeostasis," *Frontiers in Nutrition* 7 (2021): 598340, https://doi.org/10.3389/fnut.2020.598340.

52. J. Shearer and S. E. Swithers, "Artificial Sweeteners and Metabolic Dysregulation: Lessons Learned from Agriculture and the Laboratory," *Reviews in Endocrine and Metabolic Disorders* 17, no. 2 (2016): 179–86, https://doi.org/10.1007/s11154-016-9372-1.

53. Suez et al., "Artificial Sweeteners Induce Glucose Intolerance by Altering the Gut Microbiota," *Nature* 514 (2014): 181–6, https://doi.org/10.1038/nature13793.

54. N. A. Cohen and N. Maharshak, "Novel Indications for Fecal Microbial Transplantation: Update and Review of the Literature," *Digestive Diseases and Science* 62, no. 5 (2017): 1131–45, https://doi.org/10.1007/s10620-017-4535-9.

55. L. Thomas, "History of Fecal Transplant," Life Sciences, last updated February 5, 2021, accessed July 9, 2022, https://www.news-medical.net/health/History-of-Fecal-Transplant.aspx.

56. Zhang et al., "Should We Standardize the 1,700-Year-Old Fecal Microbiota Transplantation?" *The American Journal of Gastroenterology* 107, no. 11 (2012): 1755–6, https://doi.org/10.1038/ajg.2012.251.

Chapter 4

1. Imhann et al., "Proton Pump Inhibitors Affect the Gut Microbiome," *Gut* 65, no. 5 (2016): 740–8, https://doi.org/10.1136/gutjnl-2015-310376.

2. Haastrup et al., "Strategies for Discontinuation of Proton Pump Inhibitors: A Systematic Review," *Family Practice* 31, no. 6 (2014): 625–30, https://doi.org/10.1093/fampra/cmu050.

3. B. K. S. Thong, S. Ima-Nirwana, and K. Y. Chin, "Proton Pump Inhibitors and Fracture Risk: A Review of Current Evidence and Mechanisms Involved," *International Journal of Environmental Research Public Health* 16, no. 9 (2019): 1571, https://doi.org/10.3390/ijerph16091571.

4. Y. J. Choi, E. K. Ha, and S. J. Jeong, "Dietary Habits and Gastroesophageal Reflux Disease in Preschool Children," *Korean Journal of Pediatrics* 59, no. 7 (2016): 303–7, https://doi.org/10.3345/kjp.2016.59.7.303.

5. Drossman et al., "International Survey of Patients with IBS: Symptom Features and Their Severity, Health Status, Treatments, and Risk Taking to Achieve Clinical Benefit," *Journal of Clinical Gastroenterology* 43, no. 6 (2009): 541–50, https://doi.org/10.1097/MCG.0b013e318189a7f9.

6. N. Çaliskan, H. Bulut, and A. Konan. "The Effect of Warm Water Intake on Bowel Movements in the Early Postoperative Stage of Patients Having Undergone Laparoscopic Cholecystectomy: A Randomized Controlled Trial," *Gastroenterology Nursing* 39, no. 5 (2016): 340–7, https://doi.org/10.1097/SGA.0000000000000181.

7. "Chewing Your Food: Is 32 Really the Magic Number?" Healthline, October 17, 2019, accessed June 26, 2021, https://www.healthline.com/health/how-many-times-should-you-chew-your-food.

8. Cassady et al., "Mastication of Almonds: Effects of Lipid Bioaccessibility, Appetite, and Hormone Response," *The American Journal of Clinical Nutrition* 89, no. 3 (2009): 794–800, https://doi.org/10.3945/ajcn.2008.26669.

9. H. M. Staudacher and K. Whelan, "The Low FODMAP Diet: Recent Advances in Understanding its Mechanisms and Efficacy in IBS," *Gut* 66, no. 8 (2017): 1517–27, https://doi.org/10.1136/gutjnl-2017-313750.

10. "Starting the FODMAP Diet," Monash University, n.d., https://www.monashfodmap.com/ibs-central/i-have-ibs/starting-the-low-fodmap-diet/.

11. Jeitler et al., "Ayurvedic vs. Conventional Nutritional Therapy Including Low-FODMAP Diet for Patients with Irritable Bowel Syndrome: A Randomized Controlled Trial," *Frontiers in Medicine (Lausanne)* 8 (2021): 622029, https://doi.org/10.3389/fmed.2021.622029.

Chapter 5

1. C. B. Clish, "Metabolomics: An Emerging but Powerful Tool for Precision Medicine," *Cold Spring Harbor Molecular Case Studies* 1, no. 1 (2015): a000588, https://doi.org/10.1101/mcs.a000588.

2. Tang et al., "Multi-Omic Analysis of the Microbiome and Metabolome in Healthy Subjects Reveals Microbiome-Dependent Relationships Between Diet and Metabolites," *Frontiers in Genetics* 10 (2019): 454, https://doi.org/10.3389/fgene.2019.00454.

3. Q. Wu and X. Liang, "Food Therapy and Medical Diet Therapy of Traditional Chinese Medicine," *Clinical Nutrition Experimental* 18 (2018): 1–5, https://doi.org/10.1016/j.yclnex.2018.01.001.

4. "Climate Effects on Health," Centers for Disease Control and Prevention, last reviewed April 25, 2022, accessed July 14, 2022, https://www.cdc.gov/climateandhealth/effects/default.htm.

5. "Health Effects of Air Pollution," Environmental Defense Fund, accessed July 14, 2022, https://www.edf.org/health/health-impacts-air-pollution.

6. McKelvey et al., "A Biomonitoring Study of Lead, Cadmium, and Mercury in the Blood of New York City Adults [published correction appears in *Environmental Health Perspectives* 119, no. 2 (Feb 5, 2011): A57]." *Environmental Health Perspectives* 115, no. 10 (2007): 1435–41, https://doi.org/10.1289/ehp.10056.

7. Shafei et al., "The Molecular Mechanisms of Action of the Endocrine Disrupting Chemical Bisphenol A in the Development of Cancer," *Gene* 647 (2018): 235–43, https://doi.org/10.1016/j.gene.2018.01.016.

8. Stillwater et al., "Bisphenols and Risk of Breast Cancer: A Narrative Review of the Impact of Diet and Bioactive Food Components," *Frontiers in Nutrition* 7 (2020): 581388, https://doi.org/10.3389/fnut.2020.581388.

9. Rudel et al., "Food Packaging and Bisphenol A and Bis(2-Ethyhexyl) Phthalate Exposure: Findings from a Dietary Intervention," *Environmental Health Perspectives* 119, no. 7 (2011): 914–20, https://doi.org/10.1289/ehp.1003170.

10. G. E. Lloyd, ed., *Hippocratic Writings*, trans. J. Chadwick and W. N. Mann (London: Penguin; 1978).

11. Tang et al., "Does the Traditional Chinese Medicine Theory of Five Circuits and Six Qi Improve Treatment Effectiveness? A Systematic Review of Randomized Controlled Trials," *Journal of Traditional Chinese Medical Sciences* 5, no. 4 (2018): 350–60, https://doi.org/10.1016/j.jtcms.2018.12.004.

12. A. Xie, H. Huang, and F. Kong, "Relationship between Food Composition and its Cold/Hot Properties: A Statistical Study," *Journal of Agriculture and Food Research* 2 (2020): 100043, https://doi.org/10.1016/j.jafr.2020.100043.

13. Zhao Yu-xia, "Multianalysis on the Relationship between Cold and Heat Property of 176 Kinds of Common Food and Six Kinds of Nutriments Content," *Lishizhen Medicine and Materia Medica Research* (2008).

14. "The Energy of Foods in Chinese Medicine," College of Naturopathic Medicine, accessed July 14, 2022, https://www.naturopathy-uk.com/news /news-cnm-blog/blog/2020/07/16/the-energy-of-foods-in-chinese-medicine /#:~:text=Warming%20and%20cooling%20foods.

15. Wunderlich et al., "Nutritional Quality of Organic, Conventional, and Seasonally Grown Broccoli Using Vitamin C as a Marker," *The International Journal of Food Science and Nutrition* 59, no. 1 (2008): 34–45, https://doi .org/10.1080/09637480701453637.

16. "Seasonal Produce Guide," SNAP Education Connection, https://snaped.fns .usda.gov/seasonal-produce-guide.

Chapter 6

1. "How Environmental Toxins Can Impact Your Health," Cleveland Clinic Health Essentials, August 14, 2020, accessed July 16, 2022, https://health .clevelandclinic.org/how-environmental-toxins-can-impact-your-health/.

2. U. Albrecht, "Timing to Perfection: The Biology of Central and Peripheral Circadian Clocks," *Neuron* 74, no. 2 (2012): 246–60, https://doi.org/10.1016/j .neuron.2012.04.006.

3. H. Reinke and G. Asher, "Circadian Clock Control of Liver Metabolic Functions," *Gastroenterology* 150, no. 3 (2016): 574–80, https://doi.org/10 .1053/j.gastro.2015.11.043.

4. S. P. Claus, H. Guillou, and S. Ellero-Simatos, "The Gut Microbiota: A Major Player in the Toxicity of Environmental Pollutants? [published correction appears in *NPJ Biofilms Microbiomes* 3 (June 22, 2017): 17001]," *NPJ Biofilms Microbiomes* 2 (2016): 16003, https://doi.org/10.1038/npjbiofilms.2016.3.

5. K. M. Knights, A. Rowland, and J. O. Miners, "Renal Drug Metabolism in Humans: The Potential for Drug-Endobiotic Interactions Involving Cytochrome P450 (CYP) and UDP-Glucuronosyltransferase (UGT)," *The British Journal of Clinical Pharmacology* 76, no. 4 (2013): 587–602, https://doi.org/10.1111/bcp.12086.

6. S. Sharma and M. Kavuru, "Sleep and Metabolism: An Overview," *International Journal of Endocrinology* (2010): 270832, https://doi.org/10.1155/2010/270832.

7. M. L. Reed, G. R. Merriam, and A. Y. Kargi, "Adult Growth Hormone Deficiency—Benefits, Side Effects, and Risks of Growth Hormone Replacement," *Frontiers in Endocrinology (Lausanne)* 4 (2013): 64, https://doi .org/10.3389/fendo.2013.00064.

8. J. R. Davidson, H. Moldofsky, and F. A. Lue, "Growth Hormone and Cortisol Secretion in Relation to Sleep and Wakefulness," *The Journal of Psychiatry and Neuroscience* 16, no. 2 (1991): 96–102.

9. L. Thau, J. Gandhi, and S. Sharma, "Physiology, Cortisol. [Updated Sep 6, 2021]." In book: *StatPearls* [Internet] (Treasure Island, FL: StatPearls Publishing, 2022).

10. Luo et al., "Ageing, Age-Related Diseases and Oxidative Stress: What to Do Next?" *Ageing Research Reviews* 57 (2020): 100982, https://doi.org/10.1016/j.arr.2019.100982.

11. M. H. Schmidt, "The Energy Allocation Function of Sleep: A Unifying Theory of Sleep, Torpor, and Continuous Wakefulness," *Neuroscience and Biobehavioral Reviews* 47 (2014): 122–53, https://doi.org/10.1016/j.neubiorev.2014.08.001.

12. C. Iloabuchi, K. E. Innes, and U. Sambamoorthi, "Association of Sleep Quality with Telomere Length, a Marker of Cellular Aging: A Retrospective Cohort Study of Older Adults in the United States," *Sleep Health* 6, no. 4 (2020): 513–21, https://doi.org/10.1016/j.sleh.2019.12.003.

13. Fultz et al., "Coupled Electrophysiological, Hemodynamic, and Cerebrospinal Fluid Oscillations in Human Sleep," *Science* 366, no. 6465 (2019): 628–31, https://doi.org/10.1126/science.aax5440.

14. S. Makin, "Deep Sleep Gives Your Brain a Deep Clean," *Scientific American*, November 1, 2019, accessed July 16, 2022, https://www.scientificamerican.com/article/deep-sleep-gives-your-brain-a-deep-clean1/.

15. J. Lim, D. F. Dinges, "Sleep Deprivation and Vigilant Attention," *The Annals of the New York Academy of Sciences* 1129 (2008): 305–22, https://doi.org/10.1196/annals.1417.002.

16. A. Blackwelder, M. Hoskins, and L. Huber, "Effect of Inadequate Sleep on Frequent Mental Distress," *Preventing Chronic Disease* 18 (2021): E61, https://doi.org/10.5888/pcd18.200573.

17. National Institute of Diabetes and Digestive and Kidney Diseases, "Definition & Facts of NAFLD & NASH," National Institutes of Health, last reviewed April 2021, accessed July 16, 2022, https://www.niddk.nih.gov/health-information/liver-disease/nafld-nash/definition-facts#:~:text=Nonalcoholic%20fatty%20liver%20disease%20(NAFLD)%20is%20a%20condition%20in%20which,called%20alcohol%2Dassociated%20liver%20disease.

18. Zhang et al., "Rotating Night Shift Work and Non-Alcoholic Fatty Liver Disease among Steelworkers in China: A Cross-Sectional Survey," *Occupational and Environmental Medicine* 77, no. 5 (2020): 333–9, https://doi.org/10.1136/oemed-2019-106220.

19. Song et al., "Long Working Hours and Risk of Nonalcoholic Fatty Liver Disease: Korea National Health and Nutrition Examination Survey VII," *Frontiers in Endocrinology (Lausanne)* 12 (2021): 647459, https://doi.org/10.3389/fendo.2021.647459.

20. Tavares et al., "Effects of Growth Hormone Administration on Muscle Strength in Men over 50 Years Old," *International Journal of Endocrinology* (2013): 942030, https://doi.org/10.1155/2013/942030.

21. Lamon et al., "The Effect of Acute Sleep Deprivation on Skeletal Muscle Protein Synthesis and the Hormonal Environment," *Physiological Reports* 9, no. 1 (2021): e14660, https://doi.org/10.14814/phy2.14660.

22. Chennaoui et al., "How Does Sleep Help Recovery from Exercise-Induced Muscle Injuries?" *The Journal of Science and Medicine in Sport* 24, no. 10 (2021): 982–7, https://doi.org/10.1016/j.jsams.2021.05.007.

23. University of Pennsylvania School of Medicine, "Timing Meals Later at Night Can Cause Weight Gain and Impair Fat Metabolism: Findings Provide First Experimental Evidence of Prolonged Delayed Eating Versus Daytime Eating, Showing that Delayed Eating Can Also Raise Insulin, Fasting Glucose, Cholesterol, and Triglyceride Levels," *ScienceDaily*, June 2, 2017, accessed July 16, 2022, https://www.sciencedaily.com/releases/2017/06/170602143816 .htm#:~:text=impair%20fat%20metabolism-,Findings%20provide%20 first%20experimental%20evidence%20of%20prolonged%20delayed%20 eating%20versus,glucose%2C%20cholesterol%2C%20and%20triglyceride%20 levels&text=Summary%3A,more%20dangerous%20than%20you%20think.

24. Rynders et al., "Effectiveness of Intermittent Fasting and Time-Restricted Feeding Compared to Continuous Energy Restriction for Weight Loss," *Nutrients* 11, no. 10 (2019): 2442, https://doi.org/10.3390/nu11102442.

25. Adafer et al., "Food Timing, Circadian Rhythm and Chrononutrition: A Systematic Review of Time-Restricted Eating's Effects on Human Health," *Nutrients* 12, no. 12 (2020): 3770, https://doi.org/10.3390/nu12123770.

26. P. Regmi and L. K. Heilbronn, "Time-Restricted Eating: Benefits, Mechanisms, and Challenges in Translation," *iScience* 23, no. 6 (2020): 101161, https://doi .org/10.1016/j.isci.2020.101161.

27. Ravussin et al., "Early Time-Restricted Feeding Reduces Appetite and Increases Fat Oxidation But Does Not Affect Energy Expenditure in Humans," *Obesity (Silver Spring)* 27, no. 8 (2019): 1244–54, https://doi .org/10.1002/oby.22518.

28. Grundler et al., "Excretion of Heavy Metals and Glyphosate in Urine and Hair Before and After Long-Term Fasting in Humans," *Frontiers in Nutrition* 8 (2021): 708069, https://doi.org/10.3389/fnut.2021.708069.

29. Guérin et al., "Risk of Developing Colorectal Cancer and Benign Colorectal Neoplasm in Patients With Chronic Constipation," *Alimentary Pharmacology and Therapeutics* 40, no. 1 (2014): 83–92, https://doi.org/10.1111/apt.12789.

30. Savica et al., "Medical Records Documentation of Constipation Preceding Parkinson Disease: A Case-Control Study," *Neurology* 73, no. 21 (2009): 1752– 8, https://doi.org/10.1212/WNL.0b013e3181c34af5.

31. Salmoirago-Blotcher et al., "Constipation and Risk of Cardiovascular Disease among Postmenopausal Women," *The American Journal of Medicine* 124, no. 8 (2011): 714–23, https://doi.org/10.1016/j.amjmed.2011.03.026.

32. B. Ebbell, trans., *The Papyrus Ebers: The Greatest Egyptian Medical Document* (Copenhagen: Levin & Munksgaard, 1937).

33. Choe et al., "'Heat in Their Intestine': Colorectal Cancer Prevention Beliefs among Older Chinese Americans," *Ethnicity & Disease* 16, no. 1 (2006): 248–54.

34. J. M. Lattimer and M. D. Haub, "Effects of Dietary Fiber and its Components on Metabolic Health," *Nutrients* 2, no. 12 (2010): 1266–89, https://doi.org/10.3390/nu2121266.

35. Modi et al., "Implementation of a Defecation Posture Modification Device: Impact on Bowel Movement Patterns in Healthy Subjects," *Journal of Clinical Gastroenterology* 53, no. 3 (2019): 216–9, https://doi.org/10.1097/MCG.0000000000001143.

36. R. Lakhtakia, "Twist of Taste: Gastronomic Allusions in Medicine," *Medical Humanities* 40, no. 2 (2014): 117–8, https://doi.org/10.1136/medhum-2014-010522.

37. M. E. Sears, K. J. Kerr, and R. I. Bray, "Arsenic, Cadmium, Lead, and Mercury in Sweat: A Systematic Review," *Journal of Environmental and Public Health* (2012): 184745, https://doi.org/10.1155/2012/184745.

38. M. L. Hannuksela and S. Ellahham, "Benefits and Risks of Sauna Bathing," *The American Journal of Medicine* 110, no. 2 (2001): 118–26, https://doi.org/10.1016/s0002-9343(00)00671-9.

39. Laukkanen et al., "Sauna Bathing Is Associated with Reduced Cardiovascular Mortality and Improves Risk Prediction in Men and Women: A Prospective Cohort Study," *BMC Medicine* 16, no. 1 (2018): 219, https://doi.org/10.1186/s12916-018-1198-0.

40. Laukkanen et al., "Sauna Bathing Is Inversely Associated with Dementia and Alzheimer's Disease in Middle-Aged Finnish Men," *Age and Ageing* 46, no. 2 (2017): 245–9, https://doi.org/10.1093/ageing/afw212.

Chapter 7

1. Babu et al., "Rajyoga Meditation Induces Grey Matter Volume Changes in Regions that Process Reward and Happiness," *Science Reports* 10, no. 1 (2020): 16177, https://doi.org/10.1038/s41598-020-73221-x.

2. Bhasin et al., "Specific Transcriptome Changes Associated with Blood Pressure Reduction in Hypertensive Patients After Relaxation Response Training," *The Journal of Alternative and Complementary Medicine* 24, no. 5 (2018): 486–504, https://doi.org/10.1089/acm.2017.0053.

3. "12 Science-Based Benefits of Meditation," Healthline, last medically reviewed October 27, 2020, accessed July 20, 2022, https://www.healthline.com/nutrition/12-benefits-of-meditation#5.-Lengthens-attention-span.

4. Schoorlemmer et al., "Relationships between Cortisol Level, Mortality and Chronic Diseases in Older Persons," *Clinical Endocrinology (Oxford)* 71, no. 6 (2009): 779–86, https://doi.org/10.1111/j.1365-2265.2009.03552.x.

5. Vogelzangs et al., "Urinary Cortisol and Six-Year Risk of All-Cause and Cardiovascular Mortality," *The Journal of Clinical Endocrinology and Metabolism* 95, no. 11 (2010): 4959–64, https://doi.org/10.1210/jc.2010-0192.

6. Mayo Clinic Staff, "Chronic Stress Puts Your Health at Risk," Mayo Clinic, July 8, 2021, accessed July 20, 2022, https://www.mayoclinic.org/healthy-lifestyle/stress-management/in-depth/stress/art-20046037#:~:text=The%20long%2Dterm%20activation%20of,Anxiety.

7. N. Schneiderman, G. Ironson, and S. D. Siegel, "Stress and Health: Psychological, Behavioral, and Biological Determinants," *The Annual Review of Clinical Psychology* 1 (2005): 607–28, https://doi.org/10.1146/annurev .clinpsy.1.102803.144141.

8. "Inflation, War Push Stress to Alarming Levels at Two-Year COVID-19 Anniversary," American Psychological Association, March 10, 2022, accessed July 20, 2022, https://www.apa.org/news/press/releases/2022/03 /inflation-war-stress.

9. E. Won and Y. K. Kim, "Stress, the Autonomic Nervous System, and the Immune-Kynurenine Pathway in the Etiology of Depression," *Current Neuropharmacology* 14, no. 7 (2016): 665–73, https://doi.org/10.2174/15701 59x14666151208113006.

10. K. J. Ressler, "Amygdala Activity, Fear, and Anxiety: Modulation by Stress," *Biological Psychiatry* 67, no. 12 (2010): 1117–9, https://doi.org/10.1016/j.bio psych.2010.04.027.

11. P. Björntorp, "Do Stress Reactions Cause Abdominal Obesity and Comorbidities?" *Obesity Reviews* 2, no. 2 (2001): 73–86, https://doi .org/10.1046/j.1467-789x.2001.00027.x.

12. Toussaint et al., "Effectiveness of Progressive Muscle Relaxation, Deep Breathing, and Guided Imagery in Promoting Psychological and Physiological States of Relaxation," *Evidence-Based Complementary Alternative Medicine* (2021): 5924040, https://doi.org/10.1155/2021/5924040.

13. D. Chiaramonte, C. D'Adamo, and B. Morrison, "49 Integrative Approaches to Pain Management." In book: *Practical Management of Pain*, 5th ed. (Mosby, 2014), 658–68.e3, https://doi.org/10.1016/B978-0-323-08340-9.00049-9.

14. J. Nguyen and E. Brymer, "Nature-Based Guided Imagery as an Intervention for State Anxiety," *Frontiers in Psychology* 9 (2018): 1858, https://doi .org/10.3389/fpsyg.2018.01858.

15. K. Baikie and K. Wilhelm, "Emotional and Physical Health Benefits of Expressive Writing," *Advances in Psychiatric Treatment* 11, no. 5 (2005): 338– 46, https://doi.org/10.1192/apt.11.5.338.

16. Smyth et al., "Online Positive Affect Journaling in the Improvement of Mental Distress and Well-Being in General Medical Patients with Elevated Anxiety Symptoms: A Preliminary Randomized Controlled Trial," *JMIR Mental Health* 5, no. 4 (2018): e11290, https://doi.org/10.2196/11290.

17. Smyth et al., "Effects of Writing about Stressful Experiences on Symptom Reduction in Patients with Asthma or Rheumatoid Arthritis: A Randomized Trial," *JAMA* 281, no. 14 (1999): 1304–9, https://doi.org/10.1001/jama .281.14.1304.

18. M. Singh, "If You Feel Thankful, Write It Down. It's Good for Your Health," NPR, December 24, 2018, accessed July 20, 2022, https://www.npr.org /sections/health-shots/2018/12/24/678232331/if-you-feel-thankful-write -it-down-its-good-for-your-health.

19. Wood et al., "Gratitude Influences Sleep through the Mechanism of Pre-Sleep Cognitions," *The Journal of Psychosomatic Research* 66, no, 1 (2009): 43–8, https://doi.org/10.1016/j.jpsychores.2008.09.002.

20. Wood et al., "The Role of Gratitude in the Development of Social Support, Stress, and Depression: Two Longitudinal Studies," *The Journal of Research in Personality* 42, no. 4 (2008): 854–71, https://doi.org/10.1016/j.jrp.2007.11.003.

21. A. M. Wood, J. J. Froh, and A. W. Geraghty, "Gratitude and Well-Being: A Review and Theoretical Integration," *Clinical Psychology Review* 30, no. 7 (2010): 890–905, https://doi.org/10.1016/j.cpr.2010.03.005.

22. Morin et al., "Nonpharmacologic Treatment of Chronic Insomnia. An American Academy of Sleep Medicine Review," *Sleep* 22, no. 8 (1999): 1134–56, https://doi.org/10.1093/sleep/22.8.1134.

23. Parás-Bravo et al., "The Impact of Muscle Relaxation Techniques on the Quality of Life of Cancer Patients, as Measured by the FACT-G Questionnaire," *PLOS ONE* 12, no. 10 (2017): e0184147, https://doi.org/10.1371/journal.pone.0184147.

24. S. A. Mirgain and J. Singles, "Progressive Muscle Relaxation," U.S. Department of Veterans Affairs Whole Health Library, accessed July 20, 2022, https://www.va.gov/WHOLEHEALTHLIBRARY/tools/progressive-muscle-relaxation.asp.

25. O. M. Farr, C. R. Li, and C. S. Mantzoros, "Central Nervous System Regulation of Eating: Insights from Human Brain Imaging," *Metabolism* 65, no. 5 (2016): 699–713, https://doi.org/10.1016/j.metabol.2016.02.002.

26. Harvard Health Publishing, "Mindful Eating," Harvard Medical School, February 1, 2011, accessed July 20, 2022, https://www.health.harvard.edu/staying-healthy/mindful-eating.

27. López-Alarcón et al., "Mindfulness Affects Stress, Ghrelin, and BMI of Obese Children: A Clinical Trial," *Endocrine Connections* 9, no. 2 (2020): 163–72, https://doi.org/10.1530/EC-19-0461.

28. S. Nagahama et al., "Self-Reported Eating Rate and Metabolic Syndrome in Japanese People: Cross-Sectional Study," *BMJ Open* 2014;4:e005241. doi: 10.1136/bmjopen-2014-005241

29. C. E. Cherpak, "Mindful Eating: A Review of How the Stress-Digestion-Mindfulness Triad May Modulate and Improve Gastrointestinal and Digestive Function," *Integrative Medicine (Encinitas)* 18, no. 4 (2019): 48–53.

30. Carey et al., "Outcomes of a Controlled Trial with Visiting Therapy Dog Teams on Pain in Adults in an Emergency Department," *PLOS ONE* 17, no. 3 (2022): e0262599, https://doi.org/10.1371/journal.pone.0262599.

31. National Center for Emerging and Zoonotic Infectious Diseases (NCEZID), "How to Stay Healthy around Pets," Centers for Disease Control and Prevention, last reviewed April 29, 2022, accessed July 20, 2022, https://www.cdc.gov/healthypets/keeping-pets-and-people-healthy/how.html#:~:text=Most%20households%20in%20the%20United,anxiety%2C%20and%20symptoms%20of%20PTSD.

32. "The Power of Pets: Health Benefits of Human-Animal Interactions," NIH News in Health, February 2018, accessed July 20, 2022, https://newsinhealth.nih.gov/2018/02/power-pets.

33. "Health & Wellness: What about a Pet?," The Gatesworth: Seniors & Pets, https://www.thegatesworth.com/our-stories/seniors-and-pets.

Chapter 8

1. M. Carrico, "Get to Know the 8 Limbs of Yoga," *Yoga Journal,* March 23, 2021, accessed July 22, 2022, https://www.yogajournal.com/yoga-101 /spirituality/eight-limbs-of-yoga/.

2. Breit et al., "Vagus Nerve as Modulator of the Brain-Gut Axis in Psychiatric and Inflammatory Disorders," *Frontiers in Psychiatry* 9 (2018): 44, https://doi .org/10.3389/fpsyt.2018.00044.

3. A. Kamath, R. P. Urval, and A. K. Shenoy, "Effect of Alternate Nostril Breathing Exercise on Experimentally Induced Anxiety in Healthy Volunteers Using the Simulated Public Speaking Model: A Randomized Controlled Pilot Study," *Biomed Reseach International* (2017): 2450670, https://doi.org /10.1155/2017/2450670.

4. R. L. Johnson and C. G. Wilson, "A Review of Vagus Nerve Stimulation as a Therapeutic Intervention," *The Journal of Inflammation Research* 11 (2018): 203–13, https://doi.org/10.2147/JIR.S163248.

5. Harvard Health Publishing Staff, "Heart Rate Variability: How It Might Indicate Well-Being," Harvard Medical School, December 1, 2021, accessed July 22, 2022, https://www.health.harvard.edu/blog/heart-rate-variability -new-way-track-well-2017112212789.

6. van der Zwan et al., "Physical Activity, Mindfulness Meditation, or Heart Rate Variability Biofeedback for Stress Reduction: A Randomized Controlled Trial," *Applied Psychophysiology and Biofeedback* 40, no. 4 (2015): 257–268, https://doi.org/10.1007/s10484-015-9293-x.

7. K. W. Choi and H. J. Jeon, "Heart Rate Variability for the Prediction of Treatment Response in Major Depressive Disorder," *Frontiers in Psychiatry* 11 (2020): 607, https://doi.org/10.3389/fpsyt.2020.00607.

8. W. Jung, K. I. Jang, and S. H. Lee, "Heart and Brain Interaction of Psychiatric Illness: A Review Focused on Heart Rate Variability, Cognitive Function, and Quantitative Electroencephalography," *Clinical Psychopharmacology and Neuroscience* 17, no. 4 (2019): 459–74, https://doi.org/10.9758/cpn.2019.17.4.459.

9. Chang et al. "Heart Rate Variability as an Independent Predictor for 8-Year Mortality Among Chronic Hemodialysis Patients," *Scientific Reports* 10, no. 1 (2020): 881, https://doi.org/10.1038/s41598-020-57792-3.

10. de Castilho et al., "Heart Rate Variability as Predictor of Mortality in Sepsis: A Systematic Review," *PLOS ONE* 13, no. 9 (2018): e0203487, https://doi.org/10 .1371/journal.pone.0203487.

11. Hayano et al., "Survival Predictors of Heart Rate Variability after Myocardial Infarction with and without Low Left Ventricular Ejection Fraction," *Frontiers in Neuroscience* 15 (2021): 610955, https://doi.org/10.3389/fnins.2021.610955.

12. Sessa et al., "Heart Rate Variability as Predictive Factor for Sudden Cardiac Death," *Aging (Albany NY)* 10, no. 2 (2018): 166–77, https://doi.org/10.18632 /aging.101386.

13. National Center for Chronic Disease Prevention and Health Promotion, Division for Heart Disease and Stroke Prevention, "Heart Disease Facts," Centers for Disease Control and Prevention, last reviewed July 15, 2022, accessed July 22, 2022, https://www.cdc.gov/heartdisease/facts.htm #:~:text=Heart%20disease%20is%20the%20leading,groups%20in%20the%20 United%20States.&text=One%20person%20dies%20every%2036,United%20 States%20from%20cardiovascular%20disease.&text=About%20 659%2C000%20people%20in%20the,1%20in%20every%204%20deaths.

14. Dekker et al., "Low Heart Rate Variability in a 2-Minute Rhythm Strip Predicts Risk of Coronary Heart Disease and Mortality From Several Causes: The ARIC Study. Atherosclerosis Risk in Communities," *Circulation* 102, no. 11 (2000): 1239–44, https://doi.org/10.1161/01.cir.102.11.1239.

15. Goldenberg et al., "Heart Rate Variability for Risk Assessment of Myocardial Ischemia in Patients without Known Coronary Artery Disease: The HRV-DETECT (Heart Rate Variability for the Detection of Myocardial Ischemia) Study," *Journal of the American Heart Association* 8, no. 24 (2019): e014540, https://doi.org/10.1161/JAHA.119.014540.

16. J. E. Sherin and C. B. Nemeroff, "Post-Traumatic Stress Disorder: The Neurobiological Impact of Psychological Trauma," *Dialogues in Clinical Neuroscience* 13, no. 3 (2011): 263–78, https://doi.org/10.31887 /DCNS.2011.13.2/jsherin.

17. R. Yehuda and J. LeDoux, "Response Variation Following Trauma: A Translational Neuroscience Approach to Understanding PTSD," *Neuron* 56, no. 1 (2007): 19–32, https://doi.org/10.1016/j.neuron.2007.09.006.

18. Pyne et al., "Heart Rate Variability: Pre-Deployment Predictor of Post-Deployment PTSD Symptoms," *Biological Psychology* 121, Pt A (2016): 91–8, https://doi.org/10.1016/j.biopsycho.2016.10.008.

19. Kim et al., "Mind-Body Practices for Posttraumatic Stress Disorder," *The Journal of Investigative Medicine* 61, no. 5 (2013): 827–34, https://doi.org /10.2310/JIM.0b013e3182906862.

20. Lamb et al., "Non-Invasive Vagal Nerve Stimulation Effects on Hyperarousal and Autonomic State in Patients with Posttraumatic Stress Disorder and History of Mild Traumatic Brain Injury: Preliminary Evidence," *Frontiers in Medicine (Lausanne)* 4 (2017): 124, https://doi.org/10.3389/fmed.2017.00124.

21. B. Eldadah and L. Nielsen, "Research on Resilience in Stressful Times," National Institute on Aging, May 27, 2020, accessed July 22, 2022, https:// www.nia.nih.gov/research/blog/2020/05/research-resilience-stressful-times.

22. M. S. Schwartz and F. Andrasik, eds., *Biofeedback: A Practitioner's Guide* (New York: Guilford Press, 2003).

23. W. J. Cromie, "Meditation Changes Temperatures," *Harvard Gazette*, April 18, 2002, accessed July 22, 2022, https://news.harvard.edu/gazette/story/2002 /04/meditation-changes-temperatures/.

24. "Biofeedback," Mayo Clinic, accessed July 22, 2022, https://www.mayoclinic .org/tests-procedures/biofeedback/about/pac-20384664.

25. R. W. Levenson, "Blood, Sweat, and Fears: The Autonomic Architecture of Emotion," *The Annals of the New York Academy of Science* 1000, no. 1 (2003): 348–66, https://doi.org/10.1196/annals.1280.016.

26. R. Jerath and C. Beveridge, "Respiratory Rhythm, Autonomic Modulation, and the Spectrum of Emotions: The Future of Emotion Recognition and Modulation," *Frontiers in Psychology* 11 (2020): 1980, https://doi.org/10.3389/fpsyg.2020.01980.

27. Novaes et al. "Effects of Yoga Respiratory Practice (*Bhastrika pranayama*) on Anxiety, Affect, and Brain Functional Connectivity and Activity: A Randomized Controlled Trial," *Frontiers in Psychiatry* 11 (2020): 467, https://doi.org/10.3389/fpsyt.2020.00467.

Chapter 9

1. Dopico et al., "Widespread Seasonal Gene Expression Reveals Annual Differences in Human Immunity and Physiology," *Nature Communications* 6 (2015): 7000, https://doi.org/10.1038/ncomms8000.

2. Orlich et al., "Vegetarian Dietary Patterns and the Risk of Colorectal Cancers," *JAMA Internal Medicine* 175, no. 5 (2015): 767–76, https://doi.org/10.1001/jamainternmed.2015.59.

3. Brainard et al., "Health Implications of Disrupted Circadian Rhythms and the Potential for Daylight as Therapy," *Anesthesiology* 122, no. 5 (2015): 1170–5, https://doi.org/10.1097/ALN.0000000000000596.

4. Wulff et al., "Sleep and Circadian Rhythm Disruption in Psychiatric and Neurodegenerative Disease," *Nature Reviews Neuroscience* 11, no. 8 (2010): 589–99, https://doi.org/10.1038/nrn2868.

5. T. X. Phan and R. G. Malkani, "Sleep and Circadian Rhythm Disruption and stress Intersect in Alzheimer's Disease," *Neurobiology of Stress* 10 (2019): 100133, https://doi.org/10.1016/j.ynstr.2018.10.001.

6. J. R. Willis and T. Gabaldón, "The Human Oral Microbiome in Health and Disease: From Sequences to Ecosystems," *Microorganisms* 8, no. 2 (2020): 308, https://doi.org/10.3390/microorganisms8020308.

7. Woolley et al., "The Effect of Oil Pulling with Coconut Oil to Improve Dental Hygiene and Oral Health: A Systematic Review," *Heliyon* 6, no. 8 (2020): e04789, https://doi.org/10.1016/j.heliyon.2020.e04789.

8. Winnier et al., "The Comparative Evaluation of the Effects of Tongue Cleaning on Existing Plaque Levels in Children," *International Journal of Clinical Pediatric Dentistry* 6, no. 3 (2013): 188–92, https://doi.org/10.5005/jp-journals-10005-1216.

9. Peterson et al., "Modulatory Effects of Triphala and Manjistha Dietary Supplementation on Human Gut Microbiota: A Double-Blind, Randomized, Placebo-Controlled Pilot Study." *Journal of Alternative and Complementary Medicine* 26, no. 11 (2020): 1015–24, https://doi.org/10.1089/acm.2020.0148.

INDEX

A

abhyanga, 187–188, 193
acid reflux, 61, 67–69, 80
action, karma as, 8–9
acupuncture, 50
adrenal glands, 111, 182
adverse food reactions, 44–46, 199–200
aging, 115, 118–120. *See also* anti-aging
  detox
air pollution, 88
allergies (food), 44–46, 199–200
Alzheimer's disease, 116–117, 128
amygdala, 139–140
anabolism, 113–114, 115, 119–120
anti-aging detox, 109–130
  about, 109–110
  for advanced yogis, xvi–xviii
  conditions/symptoms, 113–120
  science of, 110–113
  solutions, 120–129
  tips for detoxing, 130
antibiotic use, 47, 51–52
anxiety
  doshas and, 17, 20
  intention and, 4, 5–6
  melatonin and, 36
  mind-body connection and, 139,
    142, 148–149
  panic attack and, 155–156
  root cause of, 153
aperitif, 75
appetite, 26, 64–66, 123, 146–147, 199
artificial food colors, 55–56
artificial light, 25–26, 36–37
artificial sweeteners, 56–59
asanas, 153
attachment, 8–9
autoimmune diseases, 46–48, 83–84,
  99–100
autonomic nervous system (parasym-
    pathetic and sympathetic), 135,
    136, 138, 139–140, 153–154, 156
Ayurveda
  on anxiety, 139
  on breath, 151–152
  on chronobiology, 15–20, 32
  on detoxification, 112
  detoxification ritual overview, 175–
    179. *See also* reset plan
  on digestive fire, 72, 78–80, 98
  doshas, 15–17, 20, 32, 33, 34, 187
  on metabolism, 62, 112
  on overeating and, 72
azo dyes, 56

B

bacteria. *See also* digestive health
  breast cancer and, 48–49
  gas and, 67, 70, 73
  liver detox process and, 112
  microbiome, 40, 41–43, 188–189
  morning breath and, 71
  proton pump inhibitor medication
    and, 68
bad breath, 71, 186, 204
baking soda, 54
Banyan Botanicals Blood Cleanse, 189,
  194, 197
Banyan Botanicals Chyavanprash, 198
Banyan Botanicals Total Body Cleanse,
  189, 194, 197
bedtime, 203, 204–205. *See also* sleep
beta-glucuronidase, 48–49
biofeedback, 160, 161–166
biological rhythm. *See* circadian
    rhythm
bisphenols, 89
bloated belly, 70–71. *See also* irritable
    bowel syndrome
blue light, 25, 36–37
body types. *See* doshas
bowel movements, 125–126, 189, 194,
  202–203
BPA, 89
Brahma muhrata, 33
brain
  biofeedback and, 164
  detoxification and, 111, 113,
    116–117
  intention-related neural response,
    4–7
brain fog, 116–117
breast cancer, 48–49, 89

breastfeeding, 177–178
breath, 151–170
  about, 151–153
  bad breath, 71, 186, 204
  conditions/symptoms, 155–161
  daily ritual for, 202, 203, 204
  mind-body connection and,
    153–154
  science of, 153–155
  techniques, 161–169
  tips for better breathing, 169–170
breathing rate, 164
Buddhism, 133–134
butyrate, 50

C

caffeine, 114–115, 182
cancer
  breast cancer, 48–49, 89
  detoxification and, 125, 126
  light exposure and, 25–26
  root cause of, 89
carboxymethylcellulose, 55
cardiovascular disease, 128
carrageenan, 55
catabolism, 113–114
CCF (cumin, coriander, and fennel tea)
  tea, 76, 183, 193
Center for Science in the Public Interest, 56
cerebrospinal fluid, 116
chakras, 154
change of season. *See* circadian rhythm
chewing food, 75–76, 148, 183
Chinese medicine. *See* traditional Chinese medicine
cholesterol levels, 110
chronic inflammation, 22–23, 47
chronobiology, 14–20
chyavanprash, 198
circadian rhythm, 13–38
  about, 13–14
  conditions/symptoms, 20–27
  daily ritual for, 202, 203
  detoxification and, 111–113, 114,
    118
  digestive fire and, 68–69
  digestive health and, 40
  personal routine, 29–30, 31–38
  reset ritual for, 185
  science of, 14–20
  solutions for symptoms, 27–31
Clean Fifteen™ list, 52–53
climate change, 88

cognitive restructuring, 7
cold (excess)
  conditions associated with, 94
  constitution quiz, 95–96
  food energetics and, 96–99, 101
cold water, 74–75
colorectal cancer, 125
constipation, 33, 94–95, 125–126
constitution. *See also* doshas
  determining, 95–98
  diet recommendations, 98–105
  imbalance, 91–93
  tips for, 106–107
coronary heart disease, 157–158
cortisol
  assessing levels of, 28
  catabolism and, 113–114
  circadian rhythm disruptions and,
    21, 23–26, 31
  mind-body connection, 136, 149
  muscle health and, 119–120
  personal routine for lowering levels
    of, 33, 35, 36
  stress management and, 161
  vagus nerve stimulation and, 153
COVID-19 pandemic, xix, 137–138
cravings, 65, 189
Crohn's disease, 47–49, 59
cumin, coriander, and fennel tea (CCF
  tea), 76, 183, 193
cycles. *See* circadian rhythm
cytokines, 138, 154

D

daily ritual
  about, 201
  components of, 202–205
  for optimal health, 205–206
daily routine
  bedtime, 35–38
  blueprint for, 202, 203
  for circadian rhythm synching,
    29–30, 31–38
  exercise time, 33, 34
  mealtimes, 34–35
  during reset ritual, 183–185, 192–
    194, 197
  tips, 35–38
  wake-up time, 33
dairy allergy, 44–46
dampness (excess)
  conditions associated with, 94
  constitution quiz, 95–96
  food energetics and, 96–99, 102

dementia, 116–117, 128
dental care, 185–187, 203–204
depression, 138, 142, 148–149
detoxification. *See* anti-aging detox; liver; reset plan
diaphragmatic breathing, 168–169, 202
diet. *See also* root causes
    appetite and, 26, 64–66, 123, 146–147, 199
    constitution solution, 95–105
    cravings, 65, 189
    daily ritual for, 202
    digestive fire and food choices, 84–86, 98–105
    energetics of food, 96–98
    fasting, 35, 69, 121–123
    FODMAP diet, 76–78
    food as neutral, 63
    mindful eating, 145–148, 182–183, 184, 203
    overeating, 66, 72–73, 199
    during reset ritual, 181–183, 184, 190–192, 193, 195–196, 199–200
    as root cause, 90
    seasonal diet, 104–105
    stress eating, 139–140
    tips for, 107
digestive fire, 61–81
    about, 62
    conditions/symptoms, 63–71
    diet and, 84–86, 98–105
    intermittent fasting and, 122
    science of, 62–63
    solutions for symptoms, 72–80
    tips, 80–81
digestive health, 39–60
    about, 39–41
    circadian rhythm and, 40
    conditions/symptoms, 44–49
    microbiome, 40, 41–43, 188–189
    microbiome test, 49, 50, 51
    reset ritual for, 188–189
    science of, 41–43
    solutions for symptoms, 50–59
    tips, 60
Dinges, David, 116–117
Dirty Dozen™ list, 52–53
dogs, 148–149
dopamine (feel-good neurotransmitter), 134
doshas
    circadian rhythm and, 17, 20
    influences on, 15–16
    oil massage and, 187
    personal routine and, 32, 33, 34
    quiz, 16–17
    types of, 15, 17, 32
dryness (excess)
    conditions associated with, 94
    constitution quiz, 95–96
    food energetics and, 96–99, 103
dye (food), 55–56

E

eating. *See* diet
effort, karma and, 9
elimination, 124–129, 189, 194, 202–203
emotions, 5–7, 117, 167, 179
emulsifiers, 55
endometriosis, 49
enema therapy, 59
environmental risk assessment, 88–89
enzymes (gastric juices), 67–69, 71–75, 80
epigenetics, 15
estrogen, 48–49
Evans, Arthur C., 137
exercise, 90, 185, 192–193, 197
exercise time, 33, 34, 203
external imbalance, 87–89
external stress, 135, 136
external toxins, 110

F

fall detox, 176–178
fasting, 35, 69, 121–123
fatigue, 21–23, 27–31, 46
fatty liver, 110, 111, 117–118, 129
fecal microbial transplantation (FMT), 59
feel-good neurotransmitter (dopamine), 134
fiber, 35, 59, 126
fight-or-flight mode (sympathetic system), 135, 136, 138, 139–140, 153
FODMAP diet, 76–78
food. *See* diet
food allergies, 44–46, 199–200
food coma, 66, 73
food dye, 55–56
Food Dyes: A Rainbow of Risks report, 56
forgetfulness, 116–117
future, worrying about, 133–134

G

gastric juices (enzymes), 67–69, 71–75, 80
genetics
  digestive fire and, 85
  genetic predisposition, 83, 91
  meditation retreat, 134
  organism complexity and, 41–42
  seasonal variation in gene activity, 176–177
  stem cells, xvii–xviii
GERD (gastroesophageal reflux disease), 67–68
ghrelin, 26, 65, 123
ginger tea, 69, 183
gluten allergy, 44–46
glyphosate, 53–54
good bacteria. See digestive health
gratitude, for positive outlook, 6
gratitude journal, 143
growth hormone, 113–114, 119–120
guided imagery, 142, 160, 204–205
gut. See digestive fire; digestive health

H

habits. See daily ritual
Hall, Jeffrey C., 15
happiness, 134
"happy hour" (socialization), 34
happy place, 142
haritaki, 194, 197
health, defined, xii
health intention
  about, 3–4
  karma as action, 8–9
  positive intention, 7–8
  positivity as superpower, 4–6
  positivity reprograming, 6–7
heart disease, 5, 125–126, 157–158, 177, 185
heart rate variability (HRV), 156–158, 159, 160–161, 164–165
heart rate variability monitor, 165
heartburn, 61, 67–69, 80
heat (excess)
  conditions associated with, 83–84, 93, 99–100
  constitution quiz, 95–96
  food energetics and, 96–100
heavy metals, 88–89, 124, 128
hemorrhoids, 126
herbal therapy, during reset ritual, 188–189, 194, 197, 199, 200

Hinduism, on attachment, 8
Hippocrates, 91
hope, 5
HRV (heart rate variability), 156–158, 159, 160–161, 164–165
human microbiome, 40, 41–43
Human Microbiome Project, 43
hunger, 64–66, 146–147, 199
hunger hormone (ghrelin), 26, 65, 123
hydration. See water
hygiene hypothesis, 45

I

IBD (inflammatory bowel disease), 47–48, 50, 59
IBS (irritable bowel syndrome), 59, 63–64, 70–71, 76–78
ice water, 74–75
immune system
  circadian rhythm disruption and, 21, 22–23
  gut health and, 44–49
  seasonal variation and, 176–177
inflammation (excess), 93, 99–100
inflammatory bowel disease (IBD), 47–48, 50, 59
Inner Balance, 165
insulin, 26, 30–31, 35
intention. See health intention
intermittent fasting, 35, 69, 121–123
internal clock. See circadian rhythm
internal imbalance, 87, 90
internal stress, 135, 136
internal toxins, 110
irritable bowel syndrome (IBS), 59, 63–64, 70–71, 76–78

J

Jacobson, Edmund, 143
journaling, 142–143, 194, 204–205

K

kapha dosha, 17, 187. See also doshas
karma yoga, 8–9
kaya kalpa, xvi–xviii
khichari, 191–192
kidney meridian, 139
kidneys, 112, 189

L

lactase, 67
Lactobacillus reuteri, 49
large intestine meridian, 19–20, 33
late-night eating, 122
leptin, 26, 31, 65
lifestyle
    following reset ritual, 198, 201–206
    during reset ritual, 183–185, 192–194, 195–196
light exposure, 25–26, 36–37
liver
    detoxification and, 112–113
    fatty liver, 110, 111, 117–118, 129
    reset ritual for, 182, 189
    "rhythm" of, 110–113
liver meridian, 20
loss of appetite, 64–66
low-FODMAP diet, 76–78

M

massage (oil), 187–188, 193
mealtimes, 25, 34–35, 68–69, 122, 203, 204
medical marijuana, 50
meditation, 131–133, 134, 141, 163, 204–205
melatonin, 22, 24–25, 35, 36
menopause, 48–49
menstruation, 177
meridians, 19–20, 33, 34, 139
metabolism. *See also* digestive fire
    circadian rhythm and, 26
    conditions/symptoms, 116–120
    detoxification and, 113–114
    liver and, 110–113
    solutions for symptoms, 122–124
microbiome, 40, 41–43, 188–189. *See also* digestive health
microbiome test, 49, 50, 51
migraines, 46
mind-body connection, 131–150
    about, xiii–xvi, 131–133
    breath and, 153–154, 166–167
    conditions/symptoms, 136–140, 156
    daily ritual for, 204–205
    heart rate variability and, 165
    science of, 133–135
    solutions, 140–149, 159–160, 166–169
    tips for strengthening, 149–150
mindful eating, 145–148, 182–183, 184, 203

mindfulness, for positive outlook, 6
mood and emotions, 5–7, 117, 167, 179
morning breath (bad breath), 71, 186, 204
muscles, 118–120, 164

N

NAFLD (nonalcoholic fatty liver disease), 117–118
natural cycles. *See* circadian rhythm
nature-based guided imagery, 142
negativity and negativity bias, 5–6
nervous system, 133–135
neurofeedback, 164
nightshift work, 26, 118
nirvana, steps to, 153
nonalcoholic fatty liver disease (NAFLD), 117–118
nucleus accumbens, 134
nutrition. *See* diet

O

oat-based products, 53–54
oil massage, 187–188, 193
oil pulling, 185, 204
optimal health, daily ritual for, 205–206
oral care, 185–186, 203–204
organic produce, 52–55
overeating, 66, 72–73, 199
oxidative stress, 114

P

panchakarma, xvi, xvii
pancreas, 111
panic attack, 155–156
parasympathetic system (rest-and-digest mode), 135, 138, 153–154
Parkinson's disease, 125
past and future, worrying about, 133–134
peanut allergy, 45
personal routine. *See* daily routine; doshas
pesticides, 52–55
pets, 148–149
phlebotomy, xviii
pineal gland, 36

pitta dosha, 15, 17, 20, 34, 187. *See also* doshas
PmR (progressive muscle relaxation), 143–145, 204–205
pollution, 88, 109
polycystic ovary disease (PCOS), 49, 89
polycythemia vera, xviii
polysorbate 80, 55
poop. *See* digestive health
poor appetite, 64–66
positivity
  daily ritual for, 202, 203
  intention and, 7–8
  reprograming for, 6–7
  during reset ritual, 178
  science of, 4–6
post-COVID-19 symptoms, xix
post-traumatic stress disorder (PTSD), 148, 158–161
PPIs (proton pump inhibitors), 67–68
prana (qi), 97, 152, 205
pranayama, 153, 169
prebiotics, 59
pregnancy, 177–178
present moment, 133–134
probiotics, 45, 49, 50, 51–52, 58–60
produce, 52–55
progressive muscle relaxation (PmR), 143–145, 204–205
proton pump inhibitors (PPIs), 67–68
psychomotor vigilance test (PVT), 117
PTSD, 148, 158–161

Q

qi (prana), 97, 152, 205

R

reset breaths, 169–170
reset plan, 173–200
  about, xix, 173–174
  balance, not perfection, 174–175
  detoxification ritual overview, 175–180
  frequently asked questions, 199–200
  phase 1: preparation, 179, 180–189
  phase 2: detoxification, 179–180, 189–194
  phase 3: reintroduction, 180, 195–197
  phase 4: rejuvenation, 180, 197–198
  reflection, 198
resilience, 6, 156, 161, 165–166

respiration. *See* breath
respond rather than react ("stop and think moment"), 6–7
rest-and-digest mode (parasympathetic system), 135, 138, 153–154
ritual. *See* daily ritual; reset plan
root causes, 83–107. *See also specific issues*
  about, 83–84
  health intention and, 4
  imbalances, 86–95
  science of, 84–86
  solutions for finding, 95–105
  tips for finding, 106–107
Rosbash, Michael, 15

S

Sabbagh, Marwan, 149
Sandler, Dale, 37
satiety, 146–147
satiety hormone (leptin), 26, 31, 65
sauna, 127–129, 188, 192–193
scleroderma, 83–84, 99–100
screen exposure, 24, 25, 30, 37
seasonal detoxification, 176–178
seasonal diet, 104–105
self-abhyanga technique, 187–188
serotonin, 149
sex hormones (estrogen & testosterone), 28, 48–49, 119
sleep
  bedtime, 35–38
  circadian rhythm solution, 27–31
  circadian rhythm symptoms, 22, 23–26
  daily ritual for, 204–205
  detoxification and, 114–116, 119–120
  mind-body connection and, 137, 143, 144
  as root cause, 87, 90
  wake-up time, 33
sluggishness, 66, 73, 117
small intestine meridian, 34
snacking, 69, 79
socializing time, 34
soy-based products, 53
spleen meridian, 33
spring detox, 176–178
squatting toilets, 126
stem cells, xvii–xviii
stomach acid, 67–69, 71–75. *See also* acid reflux
stomach meridian, 33

stools. *See also* digestive health
    loose, 63, 71
    sticky, 63, 71
    stool checks, 49, 50, 51
    transplant, 59
"stop and think moment" (respond
    rather than react), 6–7
stress eating, 139–140
stress management
    biofeedback for, 161–166
    conditions/symptoms of chronic
      stress, 136–140
    root cause of stress, 87, 153
    science of, 133–135
    for self-healing, xviii–xix
    techniques, 140–149, 161–162,
      166–169
suicide, 158–159
sunlight, 25
supraorganism, 43
sweating, 127–129, 164
sympathetic system (fight-or-flight
    mode), 135, 136, 138, 139–140,
    153

T

tartrazine, 56
TCM. *See* traditional Chinese medicine
tea
    cumin, coriander, and fennel, 76,
      183, 193
    for digestion, 69, 74–75, 76, 80
    ginger, 69, 183
telomeres, 115
temperature, 164
testosterone, 49, 119
therapy dogs, 148
thyroid disease, 89, 111
tongue scraping, 185–186, 204
toxins. *See* anti-aging detox; liver; reset
    plan
traditional Chinese medicine (TCM)
    on anxiety, 139
    chronobiology, 19–20, 32
    on constitution and diet, 95–105
    on constitution imbalance, 91–95
    on cycles, 15
    on yin and yang balance, 87–90
triphala powder, 189, 194, 197, 198
20-minute daily ritual, 201–206
28-day reset, 173–200. *See also* reset
    plan

U

ulcerative colitis, 50–59
urination, 127

V

vagus nerve, 153–155, 165, 168–169,
    203
vagus nerve stimulation, 154–155,
    160
vata dosha, 17, 20, 33, 139, 187. *See
    also* doshas
veterans, 158–161

W

wake-up time, 202, 203
warm liquids
    detoxification and, 183, 193–194,
      202–203
    digestive fire and, 69, 74–75, 76,
      80
water
    detoxification and, 126, 127, 183
    instead of meals, 69
    with meals, 74–75
weak digestion. *See* digestive fire
weight management
    circadian rhythm solution, 27–31
    circadian rhythm symptom, 26–27
    light exposure and, 37
    sleep and, 37–38
wine, 75

Y

yin and yang
    disease as imbalance between,
      87–90, 93–94
    food for balancing, 97–98, 99
    health as balance between, 21, 175
    stress and imbalance between, 138
yoga-based breathing exercises, 154,
    161
yogic philosophy, xiv–xvi, 153
yogurt, 58–59
Young, Michael W., 15

ACKNOWLEDGMENTS

First and foremost, I would like to express my heartfelt gratitude to my family for their unwavering support and encouragement throughout the writing of this book. Their love and patience have been my constant inspiration and motivation.

Thank you, my wonderful agents, Marc Gerald and Tess Callero at Europa Content, along with Jason Fine, for seeing the potential of *Intentional Health* and helping me manifest it into reality.

I am also deeply grateful to my editors, Lisa Cheng, Lara Asher, Monica O'Connor, Melanie Votaw, and the entire team at Hay House, who worked tirelessly to shape this manuscript into its final form. Your attention to detail, insightful feedback, and guidance have been invaluable, and I couldn't have done it without you.

Finally, I want to thank my patients for their trust, enthusiasm, and willingness to share their stories with me. Your experiences and challenges have enriched this book and helped me better understand the complexities of health and wellness. I will forever be grateful to you for allowing me to be a part of your health journey and the process of sharing this wisdom with the rest of the world.

ABOUT THE AUTHOR

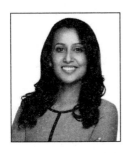 **Dr. Chiti Parikh** is a clinical professor at Weill Cornell Medicine, where she plays an active role in medical education, research, and patient care. As a board-certified internist and a holistic practitioner, she co-founded the Integrative Health and Wellbeing program at New York-Presbyterian Hospital–Weill Cornell Medicine. This program brings the best of cutting-edge Western medicine and the ancient wisdom of Eastern medicine to thousands of patients.

While growing up in India, Dr. Parikh developed an interest in the ancient traditions of yoga and meditation and started practicing at a very young age. After college, she embarked on a solo spiritual journey through Southeast Asia, where she advanced her interest in Eastern medicine. She went on to graduate with honors from Robert Wood Johnson Medical School and completed her internal medicine residency at New York-Presbyterian–Weill Cornell Medical Center.

Dr. Parikh is also trained in functional medicine, Ayurveda, acupuncture, and plant-based nutrition. As a lifelong vegetarian and practitioner of yoga, meditation, and pranayama, she practices what she preaches. Dr. Parikh has been featured on *The Dr. Oz Show*, *VICE News*, and *NBC News*, and in the *Wall Street Journal* and *Women's Health* magazine.

As a New Yorker, she understands the challenges of a hectic, stressful urban lifestyle, especially when it comes to developing healthy habits and practicing self-care. That's why she creates simple, effective, decommercialized, and decolonized wellness solutions. Her mission is to partner with her patients to create health and harmony by using her personal experience and five thousand years of science. Visit Dr. Parikh online at intentionalhealth.io.

Hay House Titles of Related Interest

YOU CAN HEAL YOUR LIFE, the movie, starring Louise Hay & Friends
(available as an online streaming video)
www.hayhouse.com/louise-movie

THE SHIFT, the movie,
starring Dr. Wayne W. Dyer
(available as an online streaming video)
www.hayhouse.com/the-shift-movie

***

*FAST LIKE A GIRL: A Woman's Guide to Using the Healing Power of Fasting
to Burn Fat, Boost Energy, and Balance Hormones,* by Dr. Mindy Pelz

*FEEDING YOU LIES: How to Unravel the Food Industry's
Playbook and Reclaim Your Health,* by Vani Hari

*HEALING ADAPTOGENS: The Definitive Guide to Using Super Herbs
and Mushrooms for Your Body's Restoration, Defense, and Performance,*
by Tero Isokauppila and Danielle Ryan Broida

All of the above are available at www.hayhouse.co.uk.

***

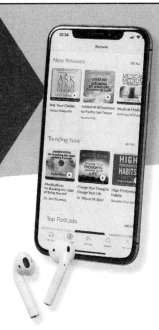

CONNECT WITH
HAY HOUSE
ONLINE

🌐 hayhouse.co.uk   **f** @hayhouse

📷 @hayhouseuk   𝕏 @hayhouseuk

▶ @hayhouseuk   ♪ @hayhouseuk

Find out all about our latest books & card decks • Be the first to know about exclusive discounts • Interact with our authors in live broadcasts • Celebrate the cycle of the seasons with us • Watch free videos from your favourite authors • Connect with like-minded souls

'*The gateways to wisdom and knowledge are always open.*'

Louise Hay